Contents

Message from the Director-General

It is with mixed feelings that I introduce *The World Health Report 1995*, for I believe no reader can turn the following pages without being struck by the scale of the global human tragedy described within them. In that sense, I am the bearer of bad news.

Producing this report, the first in an annual series, has been my personal responsibility because of the top priority given to it by the WHO Executive Board's working group on the WHO response to global change. It is not merely a statistical report, although the statistics themselves tell their own disturbing story. It is more about people's health as it affects their quality of life than about the diseases from which they suffer. As such, it is a devastating portrait of our times. It is the story of the children, adolescents, adults and elderly of this world, and the many circumstances that influence their health. In each of these age groups and also between the sexes, the report shows, there are stark and often shocking inequities in health and in access to even basic health care.

The World Health Report 1995 exposes these gaps – and advocates ways in which they can be bridged – in a form that I believe has not been attempted before. Most of all, it illustrates the growing gulf between those of us who read the report and those who are the main subject of it – the more than one billion people on this planet who live in extreme poverty.

For many of us, improvements in the quality of our lives are almost taken for granted. But at the same time vast numbers of people of all ages are suffering and dying for the want of safe water, adequate sanitation and basic medicines. This, in the last few years of the 20th century, is unacceptable.

Poverty, this report shows, is the world's deadliest disease. It wields its destructive influence at every stage of human life, and for most of its victims the only escape is an early grave. Poverty provides that too: while life expectancy is increasing in the most developed countries, it is actually shrinking in some of the poorest. For many millions of people for whom survival is a daily battle, the prospect of a longer life may seem more like a punishment than a prize.

The widening gaps between not just rich and poor, but between the poor and the poorest of all, and between those who have access to health care and those who are denied it, pose a risk that needs urgently to be recognized and countered.

The challenge is to prevent the world heading towards a health catastrophe in which many of the great achievements in health of recent decades will be thrown into reverse. There are already worrying increases in cholera, tuberculosis and plague – all diseases closely linked to poverty – while immunization rates against potentially fatal diseases are beginning to stumble backwards in some countries.

Growing inequity is literally a matter of life and death for many millions of people, since the poor pay the price of social inequality with their health. Evidence from some industrialized countries shows that a widening income gap between the rich and poor is accompanied by growing differences in mortality. On the other hand life expectancy has risen most rapidly in those developed countries where income differences have narrowed. In other words, it is the equity gap that counts. Improving the health of nations therefore

Our efforts are dedicated towards charting a better, healthier future for humanity; a future in which millions of children no longer face death in infancy nor their mothers death in childbirth; a future in which everyone has an equal chance of good health.

depends on reducing inequities both between countries, and between the rich and poor within a country.

As one of the purposes of *The World Health Report 1995* is to show what WHO is doing to help bridge the gaps, it includes a chapter on the Organization's contributions to world health – contributions that involve all its staff, whether working in the field or at regional offices or at the Geneva headquarters. It gives some idea of the wide range of activities in which WHO is involved, and some of our recent achievements. Clearly, however, the health challenges facing the world cannot be met by one organization alone.

WHO's efforts to improve health and quality of life are grounded in the firm belief that in order to bring about the necessary changes, health policies must reach beyond the health sector, while remaining rooted in the health-for-all principles of primary health care. Health is becoming a central political, social and economic issue in all countries, and health concerns must therefore be taken up at the highest political level and given due consideration in all public policies.

A better understanding is now emerging of the crucial contribution that good health makes to economic activity – enabling individuals to lead a self-fulfilling and socially and economically productive life. Perhaps the most important task of WHO is to impress upon the international community the need for political commitment to placing health and human beings at the centre of development goals. Health is not a drain on a country's resources, it is a worthwhile investment. More than that, it is the foundation on which all human endeavour rests.

Our efforts are dedicated towards charting a better, healthier future for humanity; a future in which millions of children no longer face death in infancy nor their mothers death in childbirth; a future in which everyone has an equal chance of health. The means exist; what are lacking are the commitment and resources to apply them so that the goals can be achieved. *The World Health Report 1995* is about many things, but most of all it is about people, particularly those whose plight is most desperate, and whose needs are greatest.

Their fate, like the report itself, is in your hands. I urge you not to set it lightly aside.

Hiroshi Nakajima, M.D., Ph.D.
Director-General
World Health Organization

Chapter 1
The state of world health

Introduction

The world's most ruthless killer and the greatest cause of suffering on earth is listed in the latest edition of WHO's International Classification of Diseases, an A to Z of all ailments known to medical science, under the code Z59.5. It stands for extreme poverty.

Poverty is the main reason why babies are not vaccinated, clean water and sanitation are not provided, and curative drugs and other treatments are unavailable and why mothers die in childbirth. Poverty is the main cause of reduced life expectancy, of handicap and disability, and of starvation. Poverty is a major contributor to mental illness, stress, suicide, family disintegration and substance abuse.

Poverty wields its destructive influence at every stage of human life from the moment of conception to the grave. It conspires with the most deadly and painful diseases to bring a wretched existence to all who suffer from it. During the second half of the 1980s, the number of people in the world living in extreme poverty increased, and was estimated at over 1.1 billion in 1990 – more than one-fifth of humanity.

In the time it takes to read this sentence, somewhere in the world a baby has died in its mother's arms. For that mother, the message that her neighbour's infant will live is no consolation. It does not stem her grief to know that 8 out of 10 children in the world have been vaccinated against the five major killer diseases of childhood or that globally, between 1980 and 1993, infant mortality fell by 25% while overall life expectancy increased by more than 4 years, to about 65 years.

Despite these real gains in human health, the baby still lies dead in her arms. Every year in the developing world, 12.2 million children under age 5 die, most of them from preventable causes – preventable, in many cases, for just a few US cents.

Beneath encouraging facts about decreasing mortality and increasing life expectancy, and many other unquestionable advances, lie unacceptable disparities in health – widening gaps between rich and poor, between one population group and another, between age groups and between the sexes.

For most of the people in the world today every step in life, from infancy to old age, is taken under the twin shadows of poverty and inequity, and under the double burden of suffering and disease. For many, the prospect of a longer life may seem more like a punishment than a prize.

By the end of the century we could be living in a world without poliomyelitis, a world without any new cases of leprosy, a world without deaths from neonatal tetanus and measles. But this is still 1995, and some facts of life in the world of today are deeply disturbing.

Some developing countries have less than 4 US dollars to spend per person on health care over an entire year – less than the small change many people in developed countries keep in their pockets or purses.

A person in one of the least developed countries in the world has a life expectancy of 43 years according to 1993 calculations. In one of the most developed countries it is 78 years. That is a difference of more than a third of a century. A rich, healthy man can live twice as long as a poor, sick man.

That inequity alone should stir the conscience of the world – but in some of the poorest countries the picture is getting worse. In 5 countries life expect-

> *Poverty wields its destructive influence at every stage of human life from the moment of conception to the grave. It conspires with the most deadly and painful diseases to bring a wretched existence to all who suffer from it.*

ancy is expected to decrease by the year 2000, whereas everywhere else it is increasing. In the richest countries it will reach 79 by the year 2000. In some of the poorest it will go backwards to 42 years. The gap will thus widen, from 35 years to 37, between rich and poor. By the year 2000 at least 45 countries are expected to have a life expectancy of

Fig. 1. The life expectancy marathon

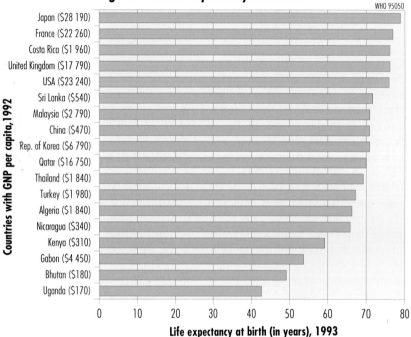

WHO 95050

under 60 years (*Fig. 1*).

In the space of a day, passengers flying from Japan to Uganda leave the country with the world's highest life expectancy – almost 79 years – and land in the one with the world's lowest – barely 42 years. A flight between France and Côte d'Ivoire takes only a few hours, but in terms of life expectancy, it spans almost 26 years. A short air trip between Florida in the USA and Haiti represents a life expectancy gap of over 19 years.

The purpose of this report is to highlight such inequities and, in a broader sense, to tackle what might appear to be simple questions, but are in reality highly complex and not amenable to simple answers.

What are the global health priorities? Which are the major diseases, the major causes of death, handicap, disabil-

ity and reduction of the quality of life? Which conditions cause most misery, although they may not be fatal? Which countries, or communities within countries, have the greatest health needs? Where should health resources be targeted?

Seeking answers to these questions is made more difficult by the poor quality or, in some instances, absence of data. The tools for measuring health status are still insufficient and even those we have can often not be employed because of lack of resources. Moreover what yardsticks should be used to measure health?

One approach is to look at mortality. Figures compiled for this report suggest that globally the biggest group of killers are infectious diseases and parasites, taking 16.4 million lives a year. These are followed by heart disease, which kills 9.7 million.

Another way to measure health is in terms of disease incidence – the number of new cases each year. Looked at this way, the biggest global problem is diarrhoea in children under age 5, with 1.8 billion episodes a year. Diarrhoeal diseases, including dysentery, claim the lives of some 3 million children a year. According to available data sexually transmitted diseases come next, with 297 million new cases per year. In third place are acute lower respiratory infections among children under age 5, such as pneumonia, with 248 million cases.

Yet another way of measuring the disease burden is in terms of prevalence – the total number of people with a given condition. According to this yardstick one of the major global health problems is goitre, with 655 million sufferers. Next comes chronic lung disease, with 600 million sufferers. But for a number of common conditions there are no measurements.

A fourth and even more difficult approach is to try to calculate the disability a disease or condition causes. The available data indicate that the biggest cause of disability across the globe is mood disorders, which affect 59 million. Other disabilities are easier to measure: blindness affects 27 million people and leprosy 2.5 million.

Table 1. Global health situation: leading causes of mortality, morbidity and disability, selected causes for which data are available, all ages, 1993 estimates[a]

Diseases/conditions[b]	Deaths Rank	Deaths Number (000)	Cases Rank	Incidence (00 000)	Cases Rank	Prevalence (00 000)	Disabled persons Rank	Disabled persons Number (permanent and long-term) (00 000)
Ischaemic heart disease	1	4 283						
Acute lower respiratory infections under age 5	2	4 110	2	2 483[e]				
Cerebrovascular disease	3	3 854						
Diarrhoea under age 5, including dysentery	4	3 010[f]	1	18 210[e]				
Chronic obstructive pulmonary disease	5	2 888			2	6 000		
Tuberculosis	6	2 709		83				
Malaria	7	2 000			5	4 000		
Falls, fires, drowning, etc.	8	1 810						
Measles	9	1 160	8	452		200		
Other heart diseases[c]	10	1 133						
Occupational injuries due to accidents		220	3	1 200				10
Chlamydial infections (sexually transmitted)			4	970[g]		1 620[g]		
Trichomoniasis			5	940[g]	7	2 360[g]		
Gonococcal infections			6	780[g]		720[g]		
Occupational diseases			7	690				
Whooping cough		360	9	431				
Genital warts			10	320				
Goitre					1	6 550		
Neurotic, stress-related and somatoform disorders					3	5 018		
Hypertensive disease					4	4 906		
Asthma					6	2 750		
Ascariasis (roundworm)		60			8	2 140		
Schistosomiasis		200			9	2 000		
Mood (affective) disorders					10	1 970	1	591
Lymphatic filariasis						1 000	2	430
Hearing loss (41 decibels and above) over age 3							3	420
Mental retardation (all types)						826	4	413
Cataract-related blindness				109			5	158
Epilepsy						298	6	149
Dementia						224	7	112
Poliomyelitis		5.5[d]		1.1			8	100
Schizophrenia						158	9	79
Obstructed labour		38		73			10	70

Leading selected causes of mortality

Leading selected causes of mortality	Deaths Rank	Deaths Number (000)
Ischaemic heart disease	1	4 283
Acute lower respiratory infections under age 5	2	4 110
Cerebrovascular disease	3	3 854
Diarrhoea under age 5, including dysentery	4	3 010[f]
Chronic obstructive pulmonary disease	5	2 888
Tuberculosis	6	2 709
Malaria	7	2 000
Falls, fires, drowning, etc.	8	1 810
Measles	9	1 160
Other heart diseases[c]	10	1 133

Leading selected causes of morbidity

Leading selected causes of morbidity	New cases annually (incidence) Rank	New cases annually (incidence) Number (00 000)	Total cases (prevalence) Rank	Total cases (prevalence) Number (00 000)
Diarrhoea under age 5, including dysentery	1	18 210[e]		
Acute lower respiratory infections under age 5	2	2 483[e]		
Occupational injuries due to accidents	3	1 200		
Chlamydial infections (sexually transmitted)	4	970[g]		1 620[g]
Trichomoniasis	5	940[g]	7	2 360[g]
Gonococcal infections	6	780[g]		720[g]
Occupational diseases	7	690		
Measles	8	452		
Whooping cough	9	431		
Genital warts	10	320		
Goitre			1	6 550
Chronic obstructive pulmonary disease			2	6 000
Neurotic, stress-related and somatoform disorders			3	5 018
Hypertensive disease			4	4 906
Malaria			5	4 000
Asthma			6	2 750
Ascariasis (roundworm)			8	2 140
Schistosomiasis			9	2 000
Mood (affective) disorders			10	1 970

Leading selected conditions/causes of disability

Leading selected conditions/causes of disability	Disabled persons (permanent and long-term) Rank	Disabled persons (permanent and long-term) Number (00 000)
Mood (affective) disorders	1	591
Lymphatic filariasis	2	430
Hearing loss (41 decibels and above) over age 3	3	420
Mental retardation (all types)	4	413
Cataract-related blindness	5	158
Epilepsy	6	149
Dementia	7	112
Poliomyelitis	8	100
Schizophrenia	9	79
Obstructed labour	10	70

a   Estimates for some diseases may contain cases that have also been included elsewhere; for example, estimates for acute lower respiratory infections and diarrhoea include those associated with measles, pertussis, malaria and HIV.
b   The ranking of diseases/conditions in this table is based on the 1993 estimates given in Table 5.
c   This category includes heart failure, nonrheumatic endocarditis, diseases of pulmonary circulation, cardiac dysrhythmias and other ill-defined conditions.
d   Estimate based on case-fatality rate for paralytic cases only.
e   Incidence estimates refer to number of episodes.
f   Deaths from dysentery estimated at 450 000.
g   Refers to maximum estimated value.
...   Data not available or not applicable.

On the basis of the data available and considered as reasonably reliable, 10 leading causes of death, illness and disability have been identified (*Table 1*). Lack of data on certain diseases has necessarily resulted in a bias that can only be progressively corrected.

The report highlights major health concerns in the world today; it does not attempt to prescribe solutions, although in some cases options are outlined. At the same time the report examines the burden of ill-health not just by disease, but also by age, as the impact of illness differs across the age spectrum. Obviously there are overlaps: malaria, for instance, affects both babies and elderly people. Where possible, however, health status has been assessed for infants and children, for adolescents, for adults and women in particular and for the elderly.

This analysis is followed by an account of what WHO is doing to bridge the gaps in health, by tackling some of the diseases and conditions that kill, disable and inflict untold suffering across the planet. Highlights of the work in different WHO regions[a] are presented. The report ends with an attempt to forecast health trends in the coming years and to chart a future for humanity – a future in which a baby will live, not die in its mother's arms.

Child health[b]

Each year the world sees some 145 million children born. For millions, their brief existence is marked by pain and disease and ends in tragically early death.

In 1993 more than 12.2 million children under the age of 5 died – a number equal to the entire populations of Norway and Sweden combined; twice as many living souls as there are in Switzerland or Hong Kong; three times the population of Ireland or New Zealand. However, 1993 also saw the number of children dying from vaccine-preventable diseases reduced by 1.3 million compared with 1985 – equal to the population of Trinidad and Tobago.

Nevertheless around 2.4 million deaths among children under age 5 are still due to vaccine-preventable diseases, particularly measles, neonatal tetanus, tuberculosis, pertussis (whooping cough), poliomyelitis and diphtheria.

World goals are to immunize at least 90% of the world's children under age 1 against these diseases by the year 2000, and also to immunize 90% of women of childbearing age. The global immunization programme, which started in its present form in 1974, has been one of the great success stories in preventive medicine – but there are worrying signs that recent gains are being eroded or even reversed by adverse social and economic conditions.

Although there were 800 000 fewer deaths from measles in 1993 than in 1985, the disease still kills about 1.2 million children each year in the developing world. In 1993 global immunization rates, per 100 surviving infants, stood at:

- 80 per 100 for poliomyelitis (3 doses);
- 79 per 100 for diphtheria-pertussis-tetanus (3 doses);
- 85 per 100 with BCG;
- 78 per 100 for measles.

However, these figures disguise deep pockets of unimmunized children. In the deprived inner-city areas of many industrialized countries, coverage is lower than in the developing world, while overall rates in Africa (at around 50%) are still significantly below the global average. Despite immunization the toll of infant and child deaths is likely to increase because of growth in the world population coupled with inability to provide optimal mother-and-child health care in many of the developing and least developed countries, where most of the deaths occur.

The gap between developed and developing world in terms of infant and child survival is one of the starkest examples of health inequity. In parts of the developed world only 6 out of 1 000 liveborns die before reaching age 5, whereas in 16 of the least developed countries the rate is over 200 per 1 000, and in one country it is 320 per 1 000. Infant mortality – deaths of children under age 1 – varies from 4.8 per 1 000

[a] See the section *Regional highlights* in *Chapter 2*, which also shows the distribution of Member States and Associate Members in the six WHO regions: Africa, Americas, Eastern Mediterranean, Europe, South-East Asia, Western Pacific.

[b] The age groupings used for the purpose of this report are: children, including infants (under age 5); school-age children and adolescents (5-19 years); adults (20-64 years); and the elderly (65 years or more). Where information cannot be assigned to one of these categories, it is given under *General health issues*.

live births to 161 – a 33-fold difference.

Of all the deaths in the developing world (adults and children combined), 31% are among children under age 5 – and most of these could have been avoided if those countries enjoyed the same health and social conditions as the world's most developed nations. Instead of more than 12 million deaths, there would have been 366 000.

In the developing world some 23% of deaths among children under age 5 occur in the first week of life, and 33% within the first month. While just under a quarter of neonatal (first week) deaths are due to prematurity and congenital defects, two-thirds of perinatal (first month) deaths are associated with the delivery itself or immediate complications and infections. In developed countries too perinatal deaths are linked to obstetric practices.

In general, while infant and child mortality rates reflect the socioeconomic development of a country, deaths during the first four weeks – and maternal deaths – are largely preventable by health care. Much of the variation between the developing and developed world in deaths among newborns can be explained by differences in antenatal care – about half of all pregnant women in the least developed countries have no antenatal care and 7 out of 10 babies are born without the help of a trained birth attendant.

Other factors contributing to perinatal and maternal mortality are the number and timing of pregnancies, and maternal malnutrition – over half the pregnant women in the developing world are anaemic (which also results in high rates of low birth weight). Nearly a quarter of newborns in the least developed countries weigh less than 2.5 kg, a rate nearly four times that in the developed countries.

Infant mortality

For most countries the infant mortality rate remains the best available overall indicator of health and development status. Although huge disparities persist, globally the infant mortality trend has been encouraging, dropping from an average of 82 per 1 000 live births in 1980 to about 62 in 1993. However, about 3 million babies in the developing world die during the first week of life.

While many countries have already reached the WHO targets for the year 2000 of infant mortality of 50 or less per 1 000 live births, and of mortality under age 5 that does not exceed 70 per 1 000 live births, at least 56 countries for which data are available have not been able to do so; and 46 of those countries are also unable to meet another key WHO target, an average life expectancy of above 60 years. In at least 15 other countries infant mortality is estimated to be above 50 per 1 000 live births. This means that in at least 71 countries with

---

Box 1. *The most deprived one in six*

A baby girl born in one of the least developed countries in 1993 can expect to live barely 44 years – 2 years more than a baby boy born in the same year. Her problems begin before birth since her mother is likely to be in poor health. If she is born in southern Asia, she has a 1 in 3 chance of being underweight, a greater chance of dying in infancy and a high probability of being malnourished throughout childhood. She has a 1 in 10 chance of dying before her first birthday and a 1 in 5 chance of dying before her fifth. In some African countries her chance of being vaccinated is less than 1 in 2. She will be brought up in inadequate housing under insanitary conditions contributing to diarrhoeal disease, cholera and tuberculosis. She will have a 1 in 3 chance of ever getting enough schooling to learn how to read and write. She may be circumcised at puberty with consequent effects on her life as a woman and a mother. She will marry in her teens and may have 7 or more children close together unless she dies in childbirth before that. Ancient traditions will prevent her from eating certain nutritious foods during her pregnancies, when she most needs building up, and dangerous practices such as using an unsterile knife to cut the umbilical cord and placing cow-dung on the stump may kill some of her babies with tetanus.

She will be in constant danger from infectious disease from contaminated water at the place where she bathes, washes clothes and collects her drinking-water. She will be chronically anaemic from poor nutrition, malaria and intestinal parasites. As well as caring for her family she will work hard in the fields, suffering from repeated attacks of fever, fatigue and infected cuts. If she survives into old age she will be exposed to the same afflictions as women in the rich countries: cardiovascular disease and cancer. To these she will succumb quickly, having no access to proper medical care and rehabilitation. She will not be able to pay anything herself: her country currently has less than $9ᶜ a year to spend on her health.

Some 24 million babies, one-sixth of the world total, were born in the least developed countries in 1993 and too many of them will grow up in miserable conditions of life and health. Equity demands that the situation of these deprived infants be improved without delay.

ᶜ Throughout this report the sign $ denotes United States dollars.

a total population of almost 2.5 billion, or almost 45% of the world population, infant mortality is 50 per 1 000 or more. The majority of these children are in Africa, and some in Asia.

The gap in infant mortality between the developed and developing world narrowed by 50% during the years 1960-1993, from 113 to 54 per 1 000 live births. At the same time the gap between least developed and developing countries widened (*Boxes 1 & 2*).

Projections suggest that in the year 2000 infant mortality in developed market-economy countries will be about 6 per 1 000, in the developing world as a whole about 60, and in least developed countries about 97. At the same time there are striking variations within regions as well as between regions. In the Americas, for example, the extremes ranged in 1993 from just over 10 in Cuba to 86 in Haiti. In Thailand the figure is just over 27, and in Bangladesh almost 107. However, higher material income need not necessarily imply a lower infant mortality or a high life expectancy at birth (*Table 2*). Several low-income countries have achieved rates that are comparable to those of richer countries.

Mortality in children under age 5

It is estimated that in 1993 global mortality among children under age 5 was 87 per 1 000 live births, i.e. for every 1 000 babies born alive, 87 would die before reaching age 5. This reflects a perceptible fall from rates of 215 during the period 1950-1955 and of 115 in 1980. However, most of the reduction is due to lower infant mortality; and it raises the question of the state of health of those children who, having survived the hazards of infancy, may subsequently be malnourished and impaired in learning and development by their fifth birthday.

Once again there are substantial differences between countries. Mortality under age 5 in the developed world was an estimated 15 per 1 000 live births in 1993, while in the developing world the figure was 97. The rate for least developed countries alone was 161.

As with infant mortality generally, the gap in mortality of children under age 5 between the developed and developing world has narrowed since 1950; but it has widened between less and least developed countries.

In the developing world, total deaths among children under age 5 in 1993 were 12.2 million, down from 13.3 million in 1985 (*Fig. 2*). Mortality was 97 per 1 000, compared with 115 in 1985. This reduction was largely due to a 35% drop in vaccine-preventable deaths as well as 13% fewer deaths from acute respiratory infections (about 8% of them from pneumonia) and 10% fewer from diarrhoea (including about 7% from diarrhoea alone).

The effects of poor nutrition

Malnutrition contributes substantially to childhood death and disease but often goes unrecognized as such. In 1990 more than 30% of the world's children under age 5 were underweight for their age. The proportion ranged from 11% of children in Latin America to 41% in Asia. The figure for Africa was 27%. This means that in 1990 some 31.6 million children in this age group were underweight in Africa, 6.4 million in Latin America and 154.8 million in Asia. In

---

Box 2. The fortunate one in eight

A baby girl born in one of the richest countries in 1993 can expect to live to the age of 82 – 6 years longer than a baby boy born in that country the same year. As she grows up she will be assured of adequate nutrition, hygienic living conditions, schooling and advanced medical care. She will receive full vaccination against all childhood diseases at the appropriate age and the proper intervals. She will probably not marry until she reaches her twenties and will then have one or two children, properly spaced and delivered in hospital after regular prenatal checkups. The greatest dangers to her health in her middle years will be the risk of an accident at home or while she is out driving, or a particularly virulent influenza epidemic. As she enters old age she will be liable to develop cardiovascular disease or cancer, but will survive the first attacks of these with little disability because of excellent medical care and rehabilitation services. She will receive good institutional care in her old age. She will spend on average, including government assistance, the equivalent of $1 540 on her health every year.

Some 17 million babies, one in eight of the world total, were born in the more developed nations in 1993 and most of them will grow up to enjoy conditions of life and health similar to those of this fortunate little girl.

the Near East the figure was 5.3 million. Although malnutrition is generally decreasing, in some areas the gain will be more than cancelled out by continuing high fertility. For example in Africa the proportion of underweight children is expected to drop from 27% in 1990 to 25% in 2005 – but the actual number will increase from 31.6 million to 39.2 million because there will be more children. In endemic areas malaria compounds the effects of poor nutrition.

The effects of some specific diseases of malnutrition have been assessed. Protein-energy malnutrition is a condition whereby people lack both energy from carbohydrates, essential protein, and vitamins and minerals. It is characterized by low birth weight if the mother is malnourished, poor growth in children and high levels of mortality in children between 12 and 24 months, and is estimated to be an underlying cause in 30% of deaths among children under age 5. While protein-energy malnutrition generally is declining, the rate is increasing in some sub-Saharan countries.

As many as 43% of children in the developing world – 230 million children – have low height for their age (i.e. stunting) and 9% – 50 million children – have low weight for height. The rate of low height for age reflects the cumulative effects of undernutrition and infections since birth or even before birth; high rates are often suggestive of bad environmental conditions and/or early malnutrition. A greater frequency of low weight for height, on the other hand, often reflects current severe undernutrition or disease. Some three-quarters of the world's malnourished children are to be found in Asia and although the overall prevalence is slowly falling, the numbers continue to rise.

Micronutrient malnutrition, estimated to affect at least 2 billion people, refers to a group of conditions caused by deficiency of essential vitamins and minerals such as vitamin A, calcium, iodine, iron and zinc. Vitamin A deficiency is still the commonest cause of preventable childhood blindness worldwide; iodine deficiency causes goitre, cretinism and brain damage; and anaemia results from insufficient iron

intake. In the developing world, more than 55% of pregnant women are anaemic. More subtle consequences of deficiencies include reduced effectiveness of the body's immune system.

Iodine deficiency disorders pose a public health problem in 118 countries, with over 1.5 billion people living in environments lacking this mineral. As a result at least 30 000 babies are stillborn each year and over 120 000 are born mentally retarded, physically stunted, deaf-mute or paralysed. Even when children are born otherwise healthy, a lack of iodine will trap them in mental dullness and apathy. The solution – iodizing salt supplies – is relatively simply and costs as little as $ 0.05 per person per year.

Table 2. Income ranges with life expectancy at birth and infant mortality rate

Income range (per capita GNP in US$) 1992	Life expectancy at birth (years) 1993	Infant mortality rate 1993
15 000 and above	70–79	5–26
10 000–14 999	72–78	7–22
5 000–9 999	63–77	9–68
1 000–4 999	51–76	10–93
500–999	45–72	24–133
100–499	43–71	27–158

Fig. 2 . Main causes of death among children under age 5 in the developing world

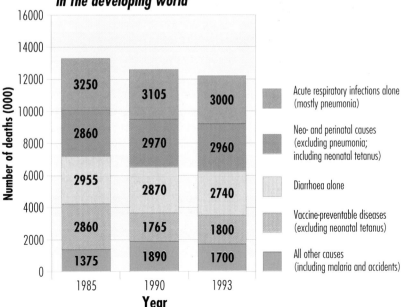

A quarter of children under age 5 in developing countries are at risk of vitamin A deficiency. Some 20% of children with this deficiency are at increased risk of death from common infections, and around 2% are blinded or suffer serious sight impairment. A number of countries have organized twice-yearly distribution by vaccination teams of vitamin A capsules to children between 6 months and 6 years. The capsules cost around $ 0.02 each.

The burden of disease

Of the more than 4 million deaths a year from acute respiratory infections in the developing world, a quarter are linked to malnutrition, and a further quarter associated with pulmonary complications of measles, pertussis (whooping cough), malaria and HIV/AIDS. Some 70% of deaths from acute respiratory infections occur before the first birthday. In 1993 one-quarter of all deaths among children under age 5, over 3 million, were due to diarrhoea and more than half of these children were malnourished. Malaria, alone or with complications, claimed nearly 1 million victims, most of them in Africa and South-East Asia (*Table 3*).

Acute respiratory infections, particularly pneumonia, were the leading causes of death and accounted for an estimated 4.1 million deaths among children under age 5 in the developing world. They are also an important cause of morbidity in children. On average, a child in both developed and developing countries has from 5 to 8 attacks annually. Although most of these attacks are mild, self-limiting episodes, they are a frequent reason for seeking health care, accounting for 30-50% of visits by children to health facilities everywhere. They are also a leading cause of disability, including deafness as a sequela of otitis media.

The incidence and severity of lung infections (pneumonia) are not spread evenly around the world. The incidence of pneumonia is almost constant in children in developed countries, varying from 3-4% a year. By contrast, the incidence in developing countries ranges between 10% and 20% but it may reach much higher levels in areas with high prevalence of risk factors such as malnutrition, low birth weight and indoor air pollution.

The problem is of enormous dimensions, but there is a workable solution. Significant and immediate reductions in mortality can be achieved by treating the underlying bacterial infections with low-cost antibiotics for a few days. More than 4 million children are dying each year – one every 8 seconds – because of a lack of appropriate antibiotics given orally for 5 days, which cost on average $0.20 per treated child.

To prevent measles and pertussis (whooping cough) it is essential to ensure that children are fully immunized. It is also important to fortify the nutritional status of children, to improve birth weight and to reduce children's exposure to indoor air pollution (*Box 3*).

Box 3. Breast-feeding

Breast-feeding is an ideal way of providing food for the healthy growth and development of infants and has a unique biological and emotional influence on the health of the mother and child. The anti-infective properties of breast milk help to protect infants against disease. Breast-feeding is associated with lower rates of ovarian and premenopausal breast cancer. It helps to reduce sepsis in newborn babies as well as chest, ear and urinary tract infections in children and gives significant protection against illness and death associated with diarrhoea in infants. Breast-feeding favours child-spacing.

Available data indicate that breast-feeding has declined in many parts of the world for a variety of social, economic and cultural reasons. With the introduction of modern technology and the adoption of new lifestyles, less importance is being attached to this traditional practice in many societies, precisely those where it is most necessary to safeguard the health of infants.

It is true that in some developed countries breast-feeding rates have shown a marked improvement. This is attributed to a combination of public education, social support and greater awareness on the part of health workers. Often, however, health services unwittingly contribute to the declining trend, either by failing to support and encourage mothers or by introducing procedures that interfere with the normal initiation of breast-feeding. Common examples of this are separating mothers from their infants at birth, giving glucose water by bottle and teat before lactation has been started, and routinely encouraging the use of breast-milk substitutes.

It is therefore essential that the staff of maternity wards and clinics for maternal and child health and family planning receive basic and in-service training on the health benefits of breast-feeding and on lactation management. All other health workers should be made fully aware of the importance of breast-feeding.

Table 3. Estimated mortality among children under age 5 in the developing world, by cause of death [a]

Cause of death	1985 Number (000)	1985 % of total	1990 Number (000)	1990 % of total	1993 Number (000)	1993 % of total	Malnutrition-associated[b] Number (000)	Malnutrition-associated[b] % of total
Total	**13 300**		**12 600**		**12 200**		**3 549**	
Acute respiratory infections	**4 730[c]**	**35.6**	**4 200[d]**	**33.3**	**4 110[e]**	**33.7**	**1 090**	**30.7**
1 ARI (mostly pneumonia)	3 250[c]	24.4	3 105[d]	24.6	3 000[e]	24.6	754	21.2
2 ARI/measles	1 085	8.2	605	4.8	640	5.2	197	5.5
3 ARI/pertussis	395	3.0	275	2.2	260	2.1	74	2.1
4 ARI/malaria	—	– –	195	1.5	190	1.6	55	1.5
5 ARI/HIV-related	—	– –	20	0.2	20	0.2	10	0.3
Neo- and perinatal	**3 640[d]**	**27.4**	**3 750[d]**	**29.8**	**3 715[e]**	**30.5**	**258**	**7.3**
6 Birth asphyxia	750	5.6	840	6.7	840	6.9	—	– –
7 Neonatal tetanus	790	5.9	555	4.4	560	4.6	—	– –
8 Congenital anomalies	395	3.0	440	3.5	440	3.6	—	– –
9 Birth trauma	375	2.8	420	3.3	420	3.4	—	– –
10 Prematurity	375	2.8	420	3.3	410	3.4	258	7.3
11 Neonatal sepsis and meningitis	175	1.3	295	2.3	290	2.4	—	– –
Diarrhoea	**3 350[f]**	**25.2**	**3 125**	**24.8**	**3 010**	**24.7**	**1 738**	**49.0**
12 Diarrhoea alone	2 955	22.2	2 870	22.8	2 740	22.5	1 582	44.6
13 Diarrhoea/measles	395	3.0	215	1.7	230	1.9	131	3.7
14 Diarrhoea/HIV-related	—	– –	40	0.3	40	0.3	25	0.7
Vaccine-preventable	**3 650**	**27.4**	**2 320**	**18.4**	**2 360**	**19.3**	**607**	**17.1**
2 ARI/measles	1 085	8.2	605	4.8	640	5.2	197	5.5
7 Neonatal tetanus	790	5.9	555	4.4	560	4.6	—	– –
15 Measles alone	495	3.7	275	2.2	290	2.4	175	4.9
16 Tuberculosis	295	2.2	295	2.3	280	2.3	—	– –
3 ARI/pertussis	395	3.0	275	2.2	260	2.1	74	2.1
13 Diarrhoea/measles	395	3.0	215	1.7	230	1.9	131	3.7
17 Pertussis alone	195	1.5	100	0.8	100	0.8	30	0.8
Measles	**1 975**	**14.8**	**1 095**	**8.7**	**1 160**	**9.5**	**503**	**14.2**
2 ARI/measles	1 085	8.2	605	4.8	640	5.2	197	5.5
15 Measles alone	495	3.7	275	2.2	290	2.4	175	4.9
13 Diarrhoea/measles	395	3.0	215	1.7	230	1.9	131	3.7
Malaria	**740**	**5.6**	**955**	**7.6**	**940**	**7.7**	**121**	**3.4**
18 Malaria alone	—	– –	635	5.0	680	5.6	66	1.9
4 ARI/malaria	—	– –	195	1.5	190	1.6	55	1.5
19 Malaria/anaemia	—	– –	125	1.0	70	0.6	—	– –
Pertussis	**590**	**4.4**	**375**	**3.0**	**360**	**3.0**	**104**	**2.9**
3 ARI/pertussis	395	3.0	275	2.2	260	2.1	74	2.1
17 Pertussis alone	195	1.5	100	0.8	100	0.8	30	0.8
Malnutrition	**—**	**– –**	**250**	**2.0**	**190**	**1.6**	**120**	**3.4**
20 Malnutrition alone	—	– –	125	1.0	120	1.0	120	3.4
19 Malaria/anaemia	—	– –	125	1.0	70	0.6	—	– –
21 **Meningitis**	**—**	**– –**	**145**	**1.2**	**100**	**0.8**	**21**	**0.6**
HIV-related	**—**	**– –**	**75**	**0.6**	**75**	**0.6**	**40**	**1.1**
14 Diarrhoea/HIV-related	—	– –	40	0.3	40	0.3	25	0.7
5 ARI/HIV-related	—	– –	20	0.2	20	0.2	10	0.3
22 HIV/others	—	– –	15	0.1	15	0.1	5	0.1
23 **Congenital syphilis**	**—**	**– –**	**195**	**1.5**	**190**	**1.6**	**—**	**– –**
24 **Accidents**	**195**	**1.5**	**195**	**1.5**	**170**	**1.4**	**—**	**– –**
25 **All other causes**	**440**	**3.3**	**200**	**1.6**	**105**	**0.9**	**46**	**1.3**

[a] Estimates as of 1 August 1994 and total deaths based on *World population prospects, 1992 revision.* New York, United Nations, 1993. First column gives item reference number.

[b] Based on the assumption that the percentage of malnutrition-asociated deaths for a given cause is constant, and that the change in the number of malnourished children is equal to changes in cause-specific deaths between 1990 and 1993.

[c] Including ARI/malaria and ARI/HIV-related deaths and 780 000 deaths from neonatal pneumonia.

[d] Including 780 000 deaths from neonatal pneumonia.

[e] Including 755 000 deaths from neonatal pneumonia.

[f] Including diarrhoea/HIV-related deaths, since they were not listed separately in 1985.

— Data not available.

– – Data not applicable.

Diarrhoeal diseases are associated with unsafe water and poor sanitation, coupled with poor food-handling practices. They are a graphic example of the synergy of poverty and lack of knowledge. Prevention and control, therefore, do not solely rest with the health services but depend on education and economic development.

Diarrhoeal diseases were responsible for around 3 million childhood deaths in the developing world in 1993. About 80% of these deaths occurred in the first two years of life. The main cause of death from acute diarrhoea is dehydration from the loss of fluids and electrolytes. Across the globe there are an estimated 1.8 billion episodes of childhood diarrhoea annually, mostly in developing countries. Each episode of diarrhoea, if not properly managed, contributes to malnutrition; when episodes are prolonged their negative impact on growth is increased. In terms of incidence, or new cases per year, this condition dwarfs all others.

Many of the deaths due to diarrhoea could also be prevented through the early replacement of fluids, usually by mouth, using whatever fluids are available in the home, and continued feeding. Children fed actively during and after diarrhoea have a better outcome; they grow normally even if they suffer repeated episodes. If children develop signs of dehydration, a special fluid containing a balanced mixture of salts (oral rehydration salts, or ORS) is needed. This fluid can be prepared in the home by mixing water with a packet of ORS.

ORS cost on average just $0.07. Thanks to local production and support from the international community, these packets are now widely available in developing countries. In some 10% of cases of dehydration, even these salts are insufficient and intravenous rehydration is required.

With multisectoral action to promote nutrition (in particular breast-feeding), food safety, education and hygienic behaviours (handwashing, proper disposal of faeces, maintaining drinking-water free from faecal contamination, thorough cooking of food) as well as through immunization against measles, the number of episodes could be substantially reduced.

Neonatal tetanus is usually caused by the introduction of tetanus spores either during delivery when the umbilical cord is cut with an unclean instrument or after delivery when the umbilical stump is "dressed" with heavily-contaminated substances, frequently as part of birth rituals. Overall the disease is fatal in 8 out of 10 cases, and it claimed the lives of an estimated 560 000 newborn babies in 1993.

The goal of eliminating neonatal tetanus has been achieved in many countries and areas, particularly through expanded immunization of women of childbearing age with tetanus toxoid. Globally, however, coverage of women is below the rates for other childhood immunizations and has risen relatively slowly, from 34% in 1990 to 45% in 1993.

Alongside immunization, the use of simple inexpensive instruments during birth can contribute substantially to tetanus reduction. Kits containing sterile equipment such as a razor blade, soap, cotton, a thread and a plastic sheet to provide a clean delivery surface have been used to very good effect in China and other parts of the world. They are usually made locally. In Nepal, for example, they are produced by a women's cooperative and sold at a very low price.

Overall, on the basis of reported coverage and estimated vaccine efficacy, WHO calculates that in 1992 *immunization* prevented 2.9 million deaths from measles, neonatal tetanus and pertussis in the developing world as well as 563 000 cases of paralytic poliomyelitis. Nevertheless there were more than 2 million deaths from measles, neonatal tetanus and pertussis, and over 114 000 cases of poliomyelitis during that year (Maps 1A & 1B). Among children born in most of the developing world, 1 in 1 000 can be expected to become lame from poliomyelitis, 4 in 1 000 to die from neonatal tetanus, 3 in 1 000 from pertussis and 1 in 100 from measles.

Since the mid-1980s there has been a striking resurgence of diphtheria in parts of eastern Europe, the Russian

> *Diarrhoeal diseases were responsible for around 3 million childhood deaths in the developing world in 1993.*

Map 1A. Global incidence of indigenous poliomyelitis, 1988

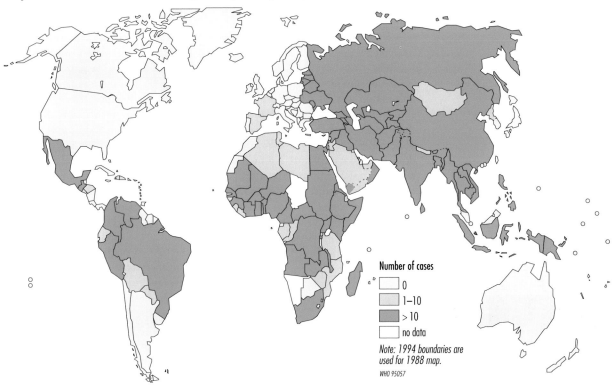

Number of cases

0

1–10

> 10

no data

Note: 1994 boundaries are
used for 1988 map.

WHO 95057

Map 1B. Global incidence of indigenous poliomyelitis, 1993

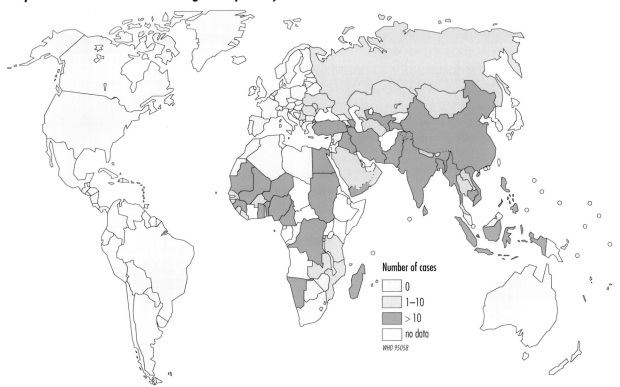

Number of cases

0

1–10

> 10

no data

WHO 95058

Federation and Ukraine. The main reasons are decreasing immunization coverage among infants and children, waning immunity in adults, population movements and an irregular supply of vaccines.

In developing countries routine immunization was introduced in the late 1970s, and coverage of infants with three doses of diphtheria toxoid reached 46% in 1985, and 79% in 1992. Recent diphtheria outbreaks in a number of countries have demonstrated a shift in the age distribution of cases to older children and adults.

Measles vaccine costs $0.14 per dose, and diphtheria-pertussis-tetanus vaccine $0.60. Because it involves only

a slight increase in cost, yellow fever vaccine has been added in the last two years to the immunization schedules of 17 of the 33 African countries at risk from this disease, and 48 countries now give routine hepatitis B vaccination to children to help prevent liver cancer.

Malaria, directly or in association with acute respiratory infections and anaemia, kills more than 1 million children a year in the developing world, accounting for about half of all malaria deaths globally, most of them in Africa. Because of the combined effects of nutritional deficiencies and malaria, many women in malarious regions are anaemic. As a result, at least 25% of babies of first pregnancies in some endemic areas have low birth weight.

Recent studies show that children's lives can be saved by bednets impregnated with insecticides. One study in Gambia found that the use of such nets reduced malaria deaths among children by 60-70%.

Ascaris, Trichuris and hookworm infections are associated with undernutrition, growth stunting and iron deficiency in children, and have an adverse effect on cognitive function in schoolchildren. It is estimated that some 204 million children aged 5-14 are affected, or 1 in 5.

Dengue also significantly affects children.

Rheumatic fever, which can cause fatal heart problems, is a major health concern in developing countries, accounting for 3 out of 10 hospital admissions.

Diabetes mellitus affects about 1 in every 1 000 children under age 15 in industrialized countries, although it appears to be rarer in developing countries – perhaps because it may be overlooked or inadequately treated. Insulin is widely available in industrialized countries, but not in the developing world because of its price there. It costs $10-12 per vial in Africa and Latin America, as compared with only $2 in western Europe. Owing to lack of insulin, many children with diabetes in developing countries die within five years of onset of the disease.

Children are bearing a huge and growing burden from the *HIV/AIDS*

Box 4. Behaviour and health

Political, economic, social, cultural, environmental and biological factors can all favour or be harmful to health. Behaviour is of importance to health either directly through learned lifestyles or indirectly in the environmental and socioeconomic context. Personal choice of behaviour can be one of several risk factors acting in combination to cause a disease (for instance poor diet, lack of exercise and smoking all contribute to cardiovascular diseases). At the same time individual and collective behaviour plays an indirect but crucial role in the prevention and control of many communicable diseases.

Lifestyle-related diseases and conditions are responsible for 70-80% of deaths in developed countries and about 40% in the developing world. Examples are cardiovascular diseases, cancer, diabetes, chronic bronchitis, obesity, malnutrition, mental and behavioural disorders, accidents and violence, alcohol and drug dependency, HIV/AIDS and other sexually transmitted diseases, vaccine-preventable infectious diseases, vectorborne and foodborne diseases, and low birth weight.

Changing people's behaviour requires an understanding of the practice and reasons that underly it as well as a clear idea of the preferred behaviour. The aim of health promotion policies and programmes should be to stimulate health awareness and responsibility and to advocate conditions which favour health.

Among the successful interventions with a significant communication and education component have been use of oral rehydration salts by mothers to prevent diarrhoeal disease in children under age 5; organization of immunization campaigns; the reduction of ischaemic heart disease in some developed countries; and improvement of nutrition. Similarly studies in developing countries have shown that mothers' knowledge of childbirth influences their participation in prenatal counselling, pregnancy behaviour and compliance with dietary recommendations. Experience of schistosomiasis control too has shown that a combination of education and community-based diagnostic and treatment services gives the best results.

The main ecological, social, economic and political actions required to create supportive environments include establishing healthy public policy with the involvement of all sectors; strengthening community participation and upgrading personnel skills; and reorienting health services towards prevention and health promotion.

pandemic, both directly as sufferers and as a result of seeing parents, siblings and other relatives die. It is estimated that by the year 2000 there will be over 5 million children infected with HIV and perhaps a further 5-10 million who have been orphaned since the pandemic began. Many AIDS orphans lack love and family support and risk becoming street children with all the attendant perils to health and emotional well-being that such a life brings.

The factors which govern transmission of the virus from infected mother to newborn baby are still far from being understood. Maternal transmission rates seem to vary across the globe, ranging from around 13% in Europe to around 30-40% in developing countries, according to some studies. The infectivity of different strains of HIV or the immune system of the mother (often weakened by malnutrition and other diseases) may be factors in the higher transmission rates in developing countries.

In Africa about 700 000 children were born to HIV-positive women in 1993 alone, of whom perhaps one-third were themselves infected. In Zambia and Zimbabwe it is calculated that AIDS will increase mortality between the ages of 0 and 4 years nearly threefold. In Thailand AIDS will increase child mortality nearly fivefold, and in Kenya and Uganda the rates will double. In short AIDS will reverse many of the hard-won improvements in child survival which have been achieved in developing countries over the past 20 years.

Health of school-age children and adolescents[d]

Across the world some 2.3 billion people, about 40% of the total population, are aged under 20. It is largely true that teenagers and young adults are biologically healthy, but young people are among the most vulnerable in terms of the diseases of society – poverty, exploitation, ignorance and risky behaviour. The least developed countries have very young and rapidly increasing populations for whom health services are not meeting adolescent needs. Education, training

and jobs for the young are not adequate. In squandering the health of its young, the world squanders its tomorrows.

The behaviour patterns established in adolescence, highly influenced by the adult world, are of immense importance to an individual's life span and to public health as a whole. The dramatic expansion of telecommunications and travel, a shrinking or in some cases disintegrating family structure, increased access to harmful substances, earlier puberty and sexual experimentation mean that adolescent behaviour has important health repercussions (*Box 4*).

Despite the difficulties they face, individual young people throughout the world contribute substantially to their

Box 5. *Health, education and nutrition*

Education of females as a driving force for better health has been extensively studied and documented. Educated women generally do not have early pregnancies, are able to space their pregnancies, have better access to information related to personal hygiene and care of their children, and make better use of health care services. Higher literacy rates among women are associated with low fertility and maternal mortality as well as with low infant mortality. Recent studies demonstrate the complexity of such relationships – for example there appears to be a link between high drop-out rates in primary schools and high prevalence of malnutrition among primary schoolchildren (*Fig. 3*). A recent study in the Indian state of Tamil Nadu, with a population of more than 60 million, showed that a midday meals programme for schoolchildren together with improvement of health care for women and their babies raised retention levels in schools, reduced child mortality, increased immunization rates – and led to a dramatic fall in infant deaths from 90 per 1 000 live births in 1984 to 57 in 1991. This in turn seems to have reduced the fertility level to 2.5 children per woman in 1991 and Tamil Nadu is now said to be on the threshold of achieving zero population growth.

Unesco's *World education report 1993* identified as a major challenge the very large numbers of youths who have never had an opportunity to receive formal education of any kind, or who have dropped out of the formal system before learning anything of value to themselves or society. The 1990 World Conference on Education for All called for innovative approaches to meeting basic learning needs, possibly utilizing the entire range of communication media available to society – popularly called the "third channel" approach. However, global use of resources for a multimedia approach is constrained by the limited communications infrastructure in many countries. Studies on the relative contributions of variables such as education, nutrition and health care and their synergistic effect on maternal and child health are being pursued by WHO to help determine the most efficient allocation of scarce resources for health.

[d] The age groupings used for the purpose of this report are: children, including infants (under age 5); school-age children and adolescents (5-19 years); adults (20-64 years); and the elderly (65 years or more). WHO defines adolescents as being between the ages of 10 and 19, and young people between the ages of 10 and 24.

families' welfare. Even in the most desperate circumstances, many young people demonstrate resilience, courage and idealism which the world cannot afford to lose. Millions belong to nongovernmental organizations (NGOs) which promote health and development and a vision of a fairer world.

Education

A blackboard and a piece of chalk can be as powerful as antibiotics and effective contraceptives. At first glance education may seem to have little to do with physical well-being and sensible fertility practices – but schooling is closely linked to health status and pregnancy rates (*Box 5 & Fig. 3*). One of the most powerful ways to promote equity, enhance development and protect health for all is to improve the education of adolescents in general and girls in particular. Education is a right to which all young people are entitled. Policies are needed to prolong minimum school-leaving ages realistically, so that girls as well as boys can benefit from modern education and training. Laws that prevent pregnant schoolgirls from attending school jeopardize their future development.

Sexual relationships and their consequences

The desire for sex and a fulfilling relationship are powerful driving forces for most young people as are pressures to engage in sexual relations; yet many are denied even basic knowledge about their own bodies or the means to protect themselves from unwanted pregnancy and sexually transmitted diseases (STDs). Pregnancy in younger women carries far higher risks of death or long-term complications than in older women, and there are severe risks in those aged 13-17. Maternal mortality rates at ages 15-19 are double the rates at 20-24, and those at ages 10-14 five times higher in some countries.

A large proportion of first marriages and first births involve adolescent women in developing countries. Recent surveys in Africa found that in 14 countries at least half the women married before the age of 18. In Niger, for example, nearly half of all women are married by the age of 15, and 2 out of 5 have at least one child by the age of 17. Studies in Latin America and the Caribbean show that 30-60% of marriages take place during adolescence. Against this background, access to information and services to prevent unwanted and too-early pregnancies is the exception rather than the rule. It is often believed that information and the provision of contraception will lead to promiscuity, whereas the evidence suggests the opposite. Moreover effective prevention of pregnancy reduces the number of abortions in young women.

Fig. 3. Health, education and nutrition

Countries with low infant mortality tend to have low fertility

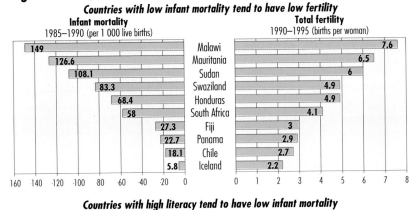

Countries with high literacy tend to have low infant mortality

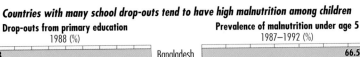

Countries with many school drop-outs tend to have high malnutrition among children

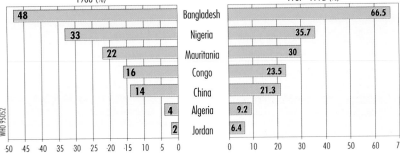

WHO 95052

Sexually transmitted diseases

STDs are most frequent in sexually active young people aged 15-24 and their high incidence is continuing. The highest rates for notifiable STDs are generally seen in the 20-24 age group, followed by those aged 15-19, then those aged 25-29. However, in most of the world the peak age of infection is lower in girls than in boys.

Although STDs are generally well treated in the developed world, adolescents are the least likely to make use of treatment services because of ignorance or fear of parental disapproval. In the developing world, facilities for treating STDs are given low priority. In addition there are worrying reports that gonorrhoea and chancroid have become resistant to inexpensive antibiotics – thereby increasing the cost of treatment in countries which can least afford it.

The long-term consequences of STDs are well established. They include infertility, pelvic inflammatory diseases, ectopic pregnancy, sepsis which can lead to death, several types of cancer particularly cervical cancer, as well as premature birth and perinatal and congenital problems.

AIDS and HIV

The hopes and lives of a generation, the breadwinners, providers and parents of the future, are in jeopardy. They include many talented citizens such as engineers, teachers, doctors, nurses and craftsmen, who could build a better world and shape the destinies of the countries they live in, and who face tragically early death.

In many countries in the developing world up to two-thirds of all new HIV infections may be occurring among 15-24 year olds. Overall it is estimated that half the global HIV infections have been in people under age 25. Up to 60% of infections in females are believed to occur by the age of 20.

The death toll from AIDS is expected to exceed 8 million by the year 2000. Most of these deaths will be in developing countries, and the remainder will be increasingly among people living in the industrialized world. AIDS will become, if it is not already, largely a disease of the poor and therefore of less interest to the rich and powerful.

The truth is that young people could be saved by using condoms. A condom costing as little as $0.03 – 3 US cents – seems a fragile barrier to hold a formidable virological foe at bay; but it is all we have, and must be used.

The unfair burden of gender

The discrimination against women that manifests itself throughout their lives begins almost from birth – in some cases even while they are still in the womb – but it becomes acute during the years of adolescence. Two centuries after the abolition of slavery in much of the world, women are still treated almost as slaves in many societies. Their chains are those of lack of education and access to fertility control, and of prejudice, discrimination and economic dependence.

As WHO's Global Commission on Women's Health forcibly points out, the adolescent girl is especially vulnerable to oppression and violence of all kinds because of her relative lack of power physically, socially and economically. She will often have lower status in the household, lower status in the workplace and less opportunity for education, training, employment and inheritance rights, all of which make for greater vulnerability. It is not just the overt acts of violence such as rape which are damaging and unquestionably underreported, but also the implicit threat of violence which may determine much of what she is obliged to do. Such violence breeds many problems, including damage to reproductive health, and has mental health consequences ranging from anxiety and sexual dysfunction to severe depression and suicide.

Tobacco, alcohol and other drugs

The seeds of unhealthy behaviour which will kill or handicap a person in adult life are laid in adolescence. Young people, because they are going through a stage of stress, experimentation and

The death toll from AIDS is expected to exceed 8 million by the year 2000.

often rebellion against parents, can be heavy users of alcohol and other drugs. In poor urban areas the sniffing of glue or paint thinners poses additional risks to health. Cigarette smoking will eventually kill 1 user in 2 and significantly shorten the lives of others. The vast majority of new smokers start in adolescence. There is growing evidence that young girls are taking up smoking. This poses an additional risk as tobacco can increase the risk of heart disease from the contraceptive pill, can cause pregnancy complications and can damage the cervix. There are high rates of smoking amongst young people in Europe,

Table 4. Smoking habits of adolescents, selected countries

Country	Year	Age group	Regular smokers (%)	
			Male	Female
France	1990	12–18	49	40
Philippines	1987	15–19	38	38
Thailand	1991	15–19	23	1

Latin America, Asia and parts of Africa (*Table 4*). Very few people take up the habit after the age of 20 or so. The sooner smoking starts, the greater is the loss of life expectancy, and the harder it is to stop. Peer group influence and advertising pressure are sowing a bitter harvest of future ill-health and early death. UNCTAD estimates that since 1988 exports of manufactured tobacco have been increasing to match the growing demand, possibly fueled by advertising.

Street children

Particularly in the megacities of the developing world, large numbers of children live and work on the streets, a high proportion without any family support. They are at high risk of malnutrition, tuberculosis, STDs including HIV and AIDS, parasite and worm infections, and skin diseases. Both sexes are highly vulnerable to drug abuse, prostitution and criminal exploitation, and in some regions street children risk summary execution from death squads. Recent estimates place their number at as many as 100 million. There may be 40 million in Latin America, 25 million in Asia and 10 million in Africa, with about 25 million in other areas including the developed world. In 1993 WHO launched an innovative project to study the links between street children and substance abuse, carrying out interviews with 550 young people in 10 cities throughout the world. The study noted regular use of alcohol and other drugs by a major proportion of street children in all cities. The most widely used substances were those which were cheap and easily available including alcohol, tobacco, cannabis, glue, solvents and pharmaceuticals. The use of cocaine, heroin, amphetamines, combinations of drugs and drug injecting was also reported. Often the lives of street children are intimately entwined with the illicit drug industry. Street children are used in the production and marketing of cocaine and the trafficking of cannabis and heroin.

Most street children describe major losses in their lives. Many have lost family members through diseases such as AIDS, natural disasters and murder. In Rio de Janeiro (Brazil) 55% of those interviewed said they had attempted to take their own lives.

Although poverty and rapid urbanization are major contributing factors to the problem of street children, many claim that physical and sexual abuse were the reasons for their leaving home. Many too are below the age of consent, do not have parents or guardians, do not know a trusted adult who could accompany them for medical treatment and do not have the necessary documentation.

There are particular problems in the provision of health and welfare services to street children with regard not only to health care but also to housing, welfare benefits, educational opportunities and employment. After being turned away from different services on many occasions, and having no adults to speak for them, the children consider it is pointless to try again even when they are in great need.

Child labour

Surveys by ILO in 1990 found that over 79 million children under the age of 15 were obliged to work. In some cases children as young as 5 years have been reported as being in paid employment. Africa and Asia dominate the data on child labour. These two regions account for 70% of the countries and 94% of the working children in a survey of more than 100 countries carried out in 1992. In Asia 15% of children aged 10-14 were working, and 22% in Africa.

Children are in particular danger from unsafe and often illegal working conditions and from exposure to hazardous chemicals, industrial acids, solvents and heavy metal fumes. Children, some as young as 6 years, labour for long hours for a half or a third of the adult wage. In the fields most work barefoot, and are thus exposed to parasites and other diseases. Many are undernourished and thus particularly vulnerable to the effects of pesticides.

In addition to paid employment, millions of children are required to do unpaid family labour, often in gruelling agricultural conditions, from hoeing and weeding to spreading pesticides and harvesting crops. Girls labour at home cleaning, cooking, fetching water and feeding domestic animals. Even small children gather firewood and parents who do not need their children's labour may hire them out to neighbouring farmers.

Accidents, violence and suicide

Between the ages of 5 and 14, injuries account for more than a fifth of deaths of boys and a seventh of deaths of girls in the developing world. In developed regions, although the number of deaths is smaller, 57% of male deaths and 43% of female deaths in this age group are due to injuries, mainly traffic accidents and drowning.

There is growing concern about the numbers of young people who die as the result of violence, and the number who are taking their own lives. Young people are increasingly victims of violence and are themselves physically aggressive to-

wards others. Every day in the USA 9 people under the age of 18 are murdered. Adolescents are twice as likely as adults to be the victims of crime, and 10 times more likely than elderly people.

There seems to be a worldwide trend of increasing violence. Poverty, unemployment, overcrowding and reduced control over the upbringing of young people are key factors. So too are drug and alcohol abuse, frequent exposure to violence on the streets and on television and for many a sense of failure, frustration and hopelessness.

That these last three emotions are widespread and profound among young people is beyond doubt, and tragically reflected in evidence that suicide rates among young people appear to be rising in both developed and developing countries more quickly than in all other age groups. In most countries suicide is second only to accidents as a leading cause of death among the young. Young men commit suicide much more often than young women who, however, attempt suicide with much greater frequency. The ratio of attempted suicide to completed suicide among adolescents has been estimated at 40 to 1 in most industrialized countries. If so many of today's young have already run out of hope, the challenge for adult society is to persuade them that life is worth living.

Health of adults

Disease patterns

In terms of disease mortality, infectious and parasitic diseases are the biggest group of killers on the planet. As far as specific causes are concerned, diseases of the circulatory system – heart attacks and stroke – are the largest single cause of death.

Globally about 51 million people of all ages died in 1993. Some 39 million deaths took place in the developing world and about 12 million in the developed. Poor countries had three times more deaths than rich ones. Some caution is necessary in interpreting mortality figures, since reliable data on causes

Suicide rates among young people appear to be rising in both developed and developing countries more quickly than in all other age groups. If so many of today's young have already run out of hope, the challenge for adult society is to persuade them that life is worth living.

Table 5. Global health situation: mortality, morbidity and disability, selected causes, all ages, 1993 estimates[a]

ICD-9 code	Diseases/conditions	Deaths (000)	Cases Prevalence (00 000)	Cases Incidence (00 000)	Disabled persons (permanent and long-term) (00 000)
	All causes	**51 000**			
	Infectious and parasitic diseases (selected), of which:	**16 445**			
480-486	Acute lower respiratory infections under age 5	4 110	...	2 483[b]	...
009	Diarrhoea under age 5, including dysentery	3 010[c]	...	18 210[b]	...
010-018	Tuberculosis	2 709	200	83	...
084	Malaria	2 000	4 000	...	...
055	Measles	1 160	...	452	...
070.2, 070.3	Hepatitis B	933	43	22	...
033	Whooping cough	360	...	431	...
320	Bacterial meningitis	210	12	...	1.9
120	Schistosomiasis	200	2 000	...	...
085	Leishmaniasis	197	127	72	...
090	Congenital syphilis	190	...	...	...
037	Tetanus	149	...	3.0	...
126	Hookworm diseases (ancylostomiasis and necatoriasis)	90	960	...	...
006	Amoebiasis (*entamoeba histolytica*)	70	480	...	...
127.0	Ascariasis (roundworm)	60	2 140	...	...
086.3-086.5	African trypanosomiasis (sleeping sickness)	55	2.7	0.6	...
086.0-086.2	American trypanosomiasis (Chagas disease)	45	170	4.0	...
125.3	Onchocerciasis (river blindness)	35	176	...	2.7
036.0	Meningitis (meningococcal)	35	3.5	...	0.5
071	Rabies	35	...	...	...
060	Yellow fever	30	...	2.0	...
061.065.4pt.	Dengue/dengue haemorrhagic fever	23	...	5.6	...
062.0	Japanese encephalitis	11	...	0.4	0.1
121pt.	Foodborne trematodes	10	...	...	...
001	Cholera (officially reported figures only)	6.8	...	3.8	...
045	Poliomyelitis	5.5[d]	...	1.1	100
032	Diphtheria	3.9	...	0.8	...
030	Leprosy	2.4	24	6.0	25
020	Plague	0.5	...	0.05	...
125pt.	Lymphatic filariasis	...	1 000	...	430
127.3	Trichuriasis (whipworm)	...	1 330	...	...
007.1	Giardiasis	...	...	5.0	...
131	Trichomoniasis	...	2 360[e]	940[e]	...
099pt.	Chlamydial infections (sexually transmitted)	...	1 620[e]	970[e]	...
078.1pt.	Genital warts	...	...	320	...
098	Gonococcal infections	...	720[e]	780[e]	...
054.1	Genital herpes	...	...	210	...
091-097	Other syphilitic infections	...	530[e]	190[e]	...
099.0	Chancroid (*haemophilus ducreyi*)	...	90[e]	90[e]	...
102,103	Endemic treponematoses	...	20	2.0	2.0
125.7	Dracunculiasis (guinea-worm disease)	...	30	20	...
279.5, 279.6	AIDS	700	10	6.2	...
795.8	*HIV (seroprevalence)*	...	*140*	...	...
	Perinatal and neonatal causes (selected), of which:	**3 180**			
768	Birth asphyxia	840	...	...	...
740-759	Congenital anomalies	660[f]	...	36	...
771.3	Neonatal tetanus	560	...	6.7	...
767	Birth trauma	420	...	...	...
764-765	Prematurity	410	...	...	...
771pt.	Neonatal sepsis and meningitis	290	...	...	...
	Maternal causes (selected), of which:	**508**			
640, 641, 666	Haemorrhage	126	...	143	3.7
647,648	Indirect causes	101	...	135	...
670	Sepsis	75	...	120	61
630-639	Abortion	67	...	199	48
642	Hypertensive disorders during pregnancy	62	...	71	0.7
643-646, 651-665, 667-669, 671-676	Other direct obstetric causes	39	...	36	...
660	Obstructed labour	38	...	73	70
	Diseases of the circulatory system (total), of which:	**9 676**			
410-414	Ischaemic heart disease	4 283	...	...	...

ICD-9 code	Diseases/conditions	Deaths (000)	Cases Prevalence (00 000)	Cases Incidence (00 000)	Disabled persons (permanent and long-term) (00 000)
430-438	Cerebrovascular disease	3,854	...	...	...
415-429	Other heart diseases[g]	1 133	...	...	...
390-398	Rheumatic fever and rheumatic heart disease	406	...	...	...
401-404	Hypertensive disease	...	4 906	...	...
	Chronic lower respiratory diseases (total), of which:	**2 888**			
491pt., 492,496	Chronic obstructive pulmonary disease	2 888	6 000	...	...
493	Asthma	...	2 750	...	...
	Malignant neoplasms/cancer (total), of which:	***6 013***	***200***	***90***	
162	Malignant neoplasm of trachea, bronchus and lung	1 035	...	...	...
151	Malignant neoplasm of stomach	734	...	...	...
153-154	Malignant neoplasm of colon and rectum	468	...	...	...
140-149	Malignant neoplasm of lip, oral cavity and pharynx	458	...	...	...
155	Malignant neoplasm of liver	367	...	...	...
174	Malignant neoplasm of female breast	358	...	...	...
150	Malignant neoplasm of oesophagus	328	...	...	...
180	Malignant neoplasm of cervix	235	...	...	...
200-202	Lymphoma	221	...	...	...
157	Malignant neoplasm of pancreas	214	...	...	...
204-208	Leukemia	207	...	...	...
185	Malignant neoplasm of prostate	182	...	...	...
188	Malignant neoplasm of bladder	135	...	...	...
183.0	Malignant neoplasm of ovary	123	...	...	...
182	Malignant neoplasm of corpus uteri	64	...	...	...
172	Malignant melanoma of skin	37	...	...	...
	Other malignant neoplasms	853	...	...	...
	External causes (total), of which:	***3 996***			
E880-E915	Falls, fires, drowning, etc.	1 810	...	...	...
E810-E829	Motor- and other road-vehicle accidents	885	...	99	...
E950-E959	Suicide	779	...	...	...
E960-E969	Homicide and violence	303	...	86	...
E916-E928	Occupational injuries due to accidents	220	...	1 200	10
	Occupational diseases	...	...	690	...
	Mental and behavioural disorders				
	Neurotic, stress-related and somatoform disorders	...	5 018	...	...
	Mood (affective) disorders	...	1 970	...	591
317-319	Mental retardation (all types)	...	826	...	413
345	Epilepsy	...	298	...	149
290	Dementia	...	224	...	112
295	Schizophrenia	...	158	...	79
	Other causes (selected), of which:	***170***			
250	Diabetes mellitus	170	600	...	...
286pt.	Haemophilia	...	3.9	0.2	...
240-242pt.	Goitre	...	6 550	...	...
282	Haemoglobinopathies	...	...	3.0	...
	Unknown causes	***8 124***			
	Disability (selected), of which:				
	Trachoma-related blindness	...	1 540	205	56
	Glaucoma-related blindness	...	201	33	51
	Cataract-related blindness	...	...	109	158
389	Hearing loss (41decibels and above) over age 3	...	...	...	420
	Alcohol and substance abuse (selected), of which:				
303	Alcohol dependence syndrome	...	...	115	...
304	Substance abuse (drug dependence syndrome)	...	...	94	...
304.3	Cannabis	...	273	...	...
304.2	Cocaine	...	94	...	...
304	Heroin	...	23	...	...

[a] Estimates for some diseases may contain cases that have also been included elsewhere; for example, estimates for acute lower respiratory infections and diarrhoea include those associated with measles, pertussis, malaria and HIV.
[b] Incidence figures refer to episodes.
[c] Deaths from dysentery are estimated at 450 000.
[d] Estimate based on case-fatality rate for paralytic cases only.
[e] Refers to maximum estimated value.
[f] Includes 440 000 deaths among children under age 5.
[g] This category includes heart failure, nonrheumatic endocarditis, diseases of pulmonary circulation, cardiac dysrythmias and other ill-defined conditions.
... Data not available or not applicable.

of death are available to WHO for only about 70 countries, which are mostly developed and account for some 40% of the world population. However, based on community studies, health service information and ad hoc surveys, an approximate distribution of deaths by cause can be made (*Table 5*).

Fig. 4. Global distribution of deaths by main causes, 1993

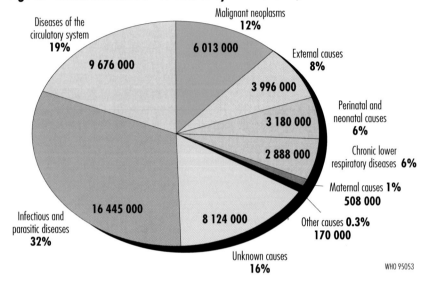

Of the estimated 51 million deaths (*Fig. 4*):

■ communicable diseases such as tuberculosis and respiratory infections as well as maternal, perinatal and neonatal causes account for about 20 million, or 40% of global deaths, and 99% of these occur in the developing world;

■ noncommunicable diseases such as cancer and heart disease account for about 19 million, or about 36% of the total, with both the developing and the developed world sharing the burden more or less equally;

■ external causes such as accidents and violence account for about 4 million, or about 8% of the total, developing countries having nearly four times the number of deaths from these causes as the developed world;

■ other and unknown causes account for the remaining 16% of global deaths.

The difference between infectious and noncommunicable diseases is very marked. One in 2 deaths in the developing world is due to communicable disease, including maternal and perinatal causes, but in the developed world 3 out of every 4 deaths are due to noncommunicable diseases, many of which are lifestyle-related (*Fig. 5*).

Fig. 5. Causes of death, 1993ᵃ

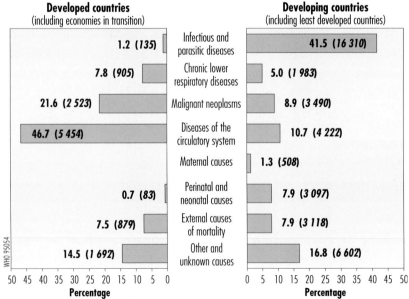

ᵃ Figures in brackets refer to the number of deaths in thousands.

The big killers

Of the 20 million deaths due to communicable diseases more than 16 million, or about 80%, are due to infectious and parasitic diseases. Tuberculosis kills about 3 million people, malaria around 2 million and hepatitis B possibly 1 million. Maternal complications claim another 508 000 lives per year.

Noncommunicable diseases are also emerging as a major cause of death in the developing world. Diseases of the circulatory system account for 10 million deaths globally of which heart disease claims more than 5 million lives and cerebrovascular disease (such as stroke) another 4 million. About 44% of the 10 million deaths from diseases of the circulatory system occur in the developing world. Cancer accounts for

6 million or 12% of deaths globally – some 58% of them in the developing world. Cancers of the airways and lungs, mostly caused by cigarette smoking, are the leading cause with 1 million deaths, followed by cancer of the stomach with over 700 000 deaths. Respiratory diseases such as chronic bronchitis kill 3 million people a year.

It is estimated that **tuberculosis** killed some 3 million people in 1993, representing more than 5% of deaths globally. There will be an estimated 8.8 million new cases in 1995. This corresponds to 52 000 deaths from the disease per week – or over 7 000 each day and over 1 000 new cases every hour of every day. Some 80% of victims are in the economically productive age group 15-49 years.

However, mortality figures, and even the number of new cases, give no real idea of the global burden of tuberculosis. Long considered a disease of the past, it has now emerged as a major public health threat and in April 1993 WHO declared it a global emergency. Some 95% of sufferers live in the developing world (*Map 2*). Tuberculosis largely affects poor people and is growing in industrialized countries.

Tuberculosis is transmitted by bacteria spread into the air when a patient with the active illness coughs or sneezes. An estimated 2 billion people carry the causative organism *Mycobacterium tuberculosis*. Most healthy people who are infected keep it in check through the strength of their immune system. The analogy of a cobra in a basket with the lid closed has been used to describe the process. When the immune system weakens through disease such as cancer or HIV or though malnutrition or old age, the lid is lifted off the basket and the cobra emerges. Once infected, a person risks developing active tuberculosis, and the risk persists throughout life. Up to 10% of those who carry the bacterium go on to develop the active form of the disease.

Drug treatment – in most cases costing as little as $13-30 per person for a six-month course – can effect a cure and stop the person being contagious. Treatment, however, requires people to take the drugs for at least six months without interruption. This is perhaps the greatest challenge to control. Many patients feel better after a few weeks and stop taking their drugs, although they are not cured and risk having a

Map 2. *Estimated tuberculosis incidence, 1990*

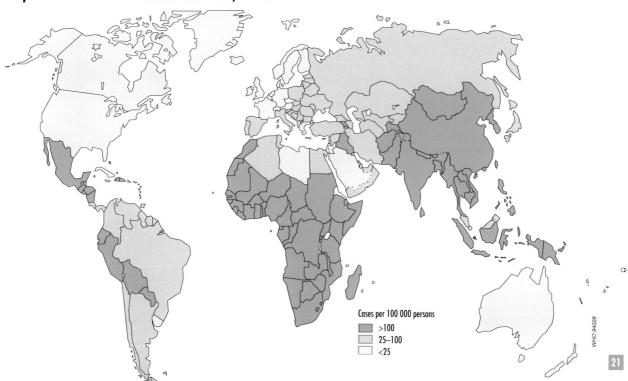

Cases per 100 000 persons

- ▓ >100
- ▒ 25–100
- ☐ <25

WHO 94028

recurrence and continuing to spread the disease. Worse, they risk developing and spreading a drug-resistant strain which is vastly more difficult and expensive to cure. Poorly managed tuberculosis programmes can thus have disastrous consequences.

BCG vaccine, developed in 1921 and still the only vaccine against the disease, is effective in protecting infants from severe forms of childhood tuberculosis. For reasons not clearly understood, it provides relatively little protection in adolescents or in adults.

HIV damages the immune system and accelerates the speed at which tuberculosis progresses from a harmless infection to a life-threatening disease – changing a process that can take years into one that happens within weeks. It may also make those who are uninfected by the tuberculosis bacterium much more vulnerable to this infection. The lethal relationship may also work the other way – tuberculosis may hasten the progress of HIV into AIDS.

The consequences of this relationship are already apparent. In sub-Saharan Africa at least 3.8 million people are infected with both tuberculosis and HIV. Asia – where 1.1 billion people suffer from tuberculosis and the number of HIV cases is rising dramatically – faces a devastating explosion of AIDS-related tuberculosis. The number of co-infected people in Asia is expected to multiply sevenfold this decade. Most will be economically productive young people aged between 20 and 49. During the next 10 years in Asia alone it is estimated that tuberculosis and AIDS together will kill more people than the entire populations of the cities of Singapore, Beijing, Yokohama and Tokyo combined.

There is every moral and practical justification for providing tuberculosis treatment in these circumstances. Treatment prevents tuberculosis being passed on. If it is denied, not only will children find themselves without one or both parents, they will discover they have been given the disease by them and are themselves at risk of an early death.

Map 3.   Countries or areas reporting cholera, 1994

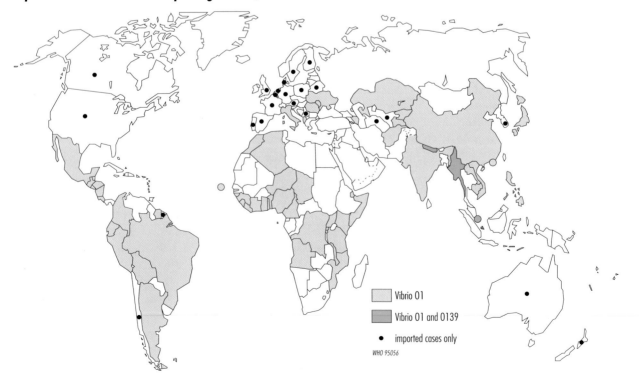

Vibrio O1

Vibrio O1 and O139

• imported cases only

WHO 95056

Currently WHO estimates that only 30% of all national tuberculosis programmes are applying the measures required to control the epidemic and that in order to undertake successful tuberculosis programmes an additional $100 million per year needs to be provided each year by donor nations to poor countries for medicines, microscopes and a modest infrastructure. Meanwhile low-cost drugs which are almost 100% effective sit on shelves unused.

Cholera has become endemic in many countries in Africa, Asia and Latin America (*Map 3*). In 1993 there were 377 000 new cases reported and 6 800 deaths. The global case fatality rate is currently about 1.8%, which is much lower than previous values due to simple, cheap and effective case management promoted by WHO. The total number of cases officially reported to WHO declined from a peak of around 600 000 in 1991. Nevertheless the numbers of cases and deaths remain at far higher levels than those reported earlier. The largest decline in incidence between 1992 and 1993 was seen in the Americas, which since 1991 had been the source of most reports. Africa continues to report a considerable number of cases and deaths, accounting for about 25% of the global total in 1993 (see also *Box 6*). In Asia officially reported cases more than doubled between 1992 and 1993, with a large outbreak in war-torn Afghanistan accounting for a substantial part of the increase.

Complicating the situation in Asia was the emergence in late 1992 of a new causative organism, designated *Vibrio cholerae O139* (Bengal). This strain has spread very rapidly through Bangladesh, China, India, Malaysia, Nepal and Pakistan and has caused unusually high mortality, even in adults. Previous exposure to *Vibrio cholerae O1* (El Tor), the classical cholera strain since the mid-1960s, does not provide protective immunity against the new organism.

Malaria is by far the most important tropical parasitic disease, causing immense suffering and loss of life. The enormous toll of lives and of days of labour lost, and the costs of treatment, make malaria a major social and economic burden in developing countries. The estimated direct and indirect cost of the disease in Africa alone is expected to have reached $1.8 billion by 1995.

Malaria is caused by four species of protozoal parasites of the genus *Plasmodium*. Of these, *P.falciparum* accounts for most of the infections in Africa and for over a third of infections in the rest of the world. Falciparum malaria is the most dangerous form of the disease, sometimes progressing to cerebral oedema, coma and death.

There are an estimated 2 million deaths a year, 90% in Africa and the vast majority among young children. Outside Africa two-thirds of the reported cases are concentrated in only 6 countries, namely in decreasing order: India, Brazil, Sri Lanka, Afghanistan, Viet Nam and Colombia. Around the world more than 2 billion people are threatened.

The global malaria control strategy adopted in 1992 emphasises early diagnosis and treatment of the disease with effective antimalarial drugs, selective application of preventive measures including vector control where the results are cost-effective and sustainable, the detection, prevention and control of epidemics and the continuous review of the local malaria situation so that control measures can be adapted as necessary.

Box 6. Cholera outbreak in Goma (Zaire)

July 1994 saw a large and dramatic outbreak of cholera in camps in Goma (Zaire). The rapid influx of an estimated 700 000 to 1 million Rwandan refugees to the city of Goma and surrounding areas resulted in massive overcrowding without basic sanitation or safe water, creating ideal conditions for rapid spread of the disease. On the basis of epidemiological surveillance, it was estimated that 70 000 cases of diarrhoeal disease, including many cholera cases, occurred in Goma between 20 July and 12 August 1994.

Despite the suddenness and size of the outbreak, case fatality decreased from 24% during the first days of the epidemic to 3-5% with the establishment of rehydration units and the distribution of safe water.

There was a strong response to the outbreak by the international community. WHO played a crucial role in providing technical advice on cholera and dysentery control to relief agencies working in the refugee camps, thus ensuring a concerted international effort. Teams were sent from WHO headquarters and the Regional Office for Africa to assist in the work.

Although the geographical area affected by the illness has shrunk dramatically over the past 50 years, gains are being eroded (*Maps 4A & 4B*). Control is becoming increasingly difficult, manifestations of the disease appear to be more severe than in the past, and there is a growing problem of drug resistance.

Malaria is treated with a number of drugs, used either together or singly depending on the resistance of the parasite. Treatment costs are in the range of $3.50-12.50 per person per year. Chloroquine was until recently the drug of choice in Africa, but resistance is beginning to compromise its use there. New drugs have been developed, but resistance to some of these is being reported at an alarming rate. Moreover improvements in malaria control face formidable challenges in many areas where there is a lack of basic health care infrastructure. Three main types of vaccine that may contribute to the control of malaria are currently under development as described in *Chapter 2*. Recent findings indicate that there are good prospects of having a vaccine before the end of the decade.

The spread of malaria is linked to activities such as road building, mining, logging and new agricultural and irrigation projects. It is a particular problem in "frontier" areas such as Amazonia. Malaria is not only a devastating disease for the individual, but a social condition closely related to economic development and in many cases an important obstacle to development.

Other communicable diseases

Dengue and **dengue haemorrhagic fever** are now the most important and rapidly rising arbovirus infections in the world. They are mosquito-borne diseases related to yellow fever. There are four distinct dengue viruses, with no cross-immunity between them, so that an individual who has recovered from one remains susceptible to the other three. It is even thought that a previous infection makes people more susceptible to serious complications or to subsequent infections. The breeding habits of the main mosquito vector, *Aedes aegypti*, are

closely related to poor sanitation or overcrowding and incorrect water storage.

Although debilitating symptoms and death are inflicted on all social strata, dengue frequently affects the very young and the elderly. There are millions of cases annually, with more than 500 000 people needing hospital treatment, and thousands of deaths. Dengue has recently caused massive epidemics in Africa, the Americas, Asia, the Pacific islands and in some countries of the Eastern Mediterranean. From 1955 to 1970 only 9 countries reported epidemics of dengue haemorrhagic fever. Between 1970 and 1993, however, a further 28 countries were affected.

If diagnosed and treated early, mortality from dengue haemorrhagic fever is less than 5%; otherwise it can be 30%. But in many countries clinicians do not recognize symptoms, laboratories are not equipped for diagnosis, diagnostic kits are not available and vector control programmes are insufficient.

The ancient scourge of **leprosy** still causes 600 000 new cases a year. Between 2 and 3 million people are disabled by the disease, including those who have been cured but crippled in some way prior to treatment. It affects 79 countries but the majority of victims are in India, Myanmar and Brazil (*Maps 5A & 5B*).

The route of infection is thought to be coughing and sneezing, but transmission is very inefficient. Of those infected with the slow-growing leprosy bacillus, few develop the disease. Of the estimated 2.4 million sufferers, 1.7 million are known and receiving treatment.

Dapsone, the first really effective drug against leprosy, was used on a large scale from the 1950s onwards, but widespread resistance soon developed. Later, new effective drugs were synthesized. Use of a combination of three different drugs was shown to be very effective, because the likelihood of a bacterium being resistant to all the three at the same time is practically nil. This multidrug therapy developed and promoted by WHO is successful in curing the disease and making patients noninfectious. If such treatment can be made available to all patients, there is

The ancient scourge of leprosy still causes 600 000 new cases a year. Between 2 and 3 million people are disabled by the disease.

Map 4A. Geographical distribution of malaria before 1946

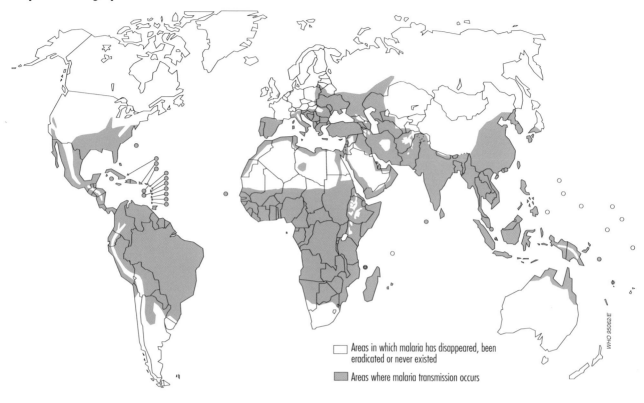

☐ Areas in which malaria has disappeared, been eradicated or never existed

▩ Areas where malaria transmission occurs

WHO 95062/E

Map 4B. Epidemiological status of malaria, 1994

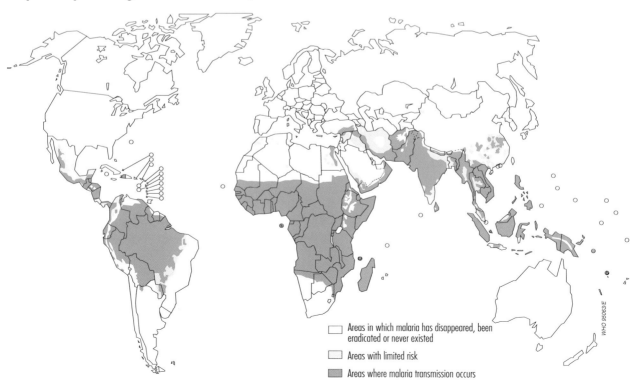

☐ Areas in which malaria has disappeared, been eradicated or never existed

☐ Areas with limited risk

▩ Areas where malaria transmission occurs

WHO 95063/E

Map 5A. Registered leprosy cases in the world, 1985

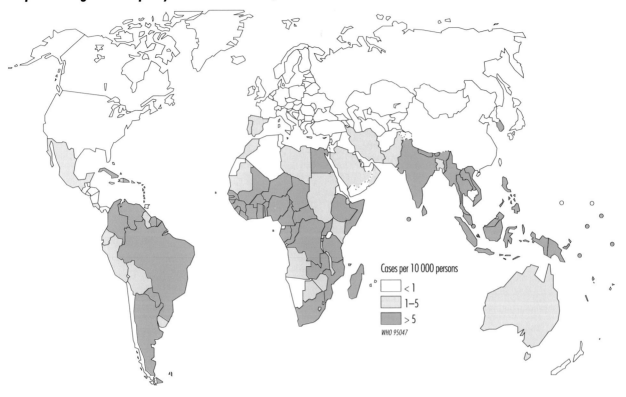

Cases per 10 000 persons

☐ < 1
▨ 1–5
▩ > 5

WHO 95047

Map 5B. Registered leprosy cases in the world, 1994

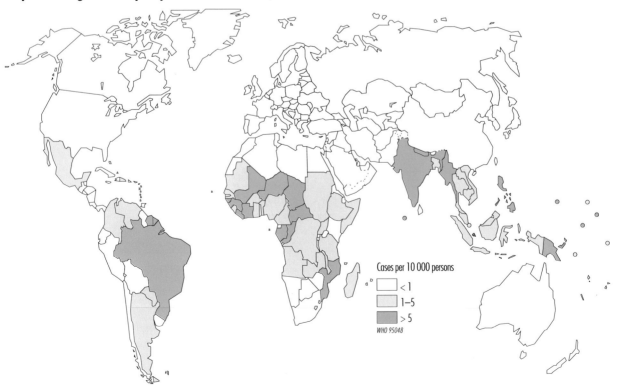

Cases per 10 000 persons

☐ < 1
▨ 1–5
▩ > 5

WHO 95048

hope that the WHO target of eliminating leprosy as a public health problem can be reached.

Onchocerciasis (river blindness) infects 18 million people in 34 countries mainly in western Africa, but also in Yemen and Latin America. Some 300 000 people have been blinded by the disease. In the west African savanna, where the parasite strain is most pathogenic to the eye, 1 in 10 people risked blindness before the disease was brought under control. In addition to causing around 40 000 new cases of blindness each year, it also provokes severe itching as well as disfiguring skin disease. WHO has shown that one tablet a year of the drug ivermectin can prevent the disease. The drug has been provided free of charge to the programme by its manufacturer Merck & Co, and is currently being taken by more than 2.5 million people a year. However, many of the most affected communities are located in remote areas and are hard to reach. As a result, the disease remains a major health concern in Cameroon and Nigeria among others.

Dracunculiasis (guinea-worm disease) causes dreadful suffering and disability among the world's most deprived people. Nine out of ten people living in the depressed areas of Africa south of the Sahara and of the Indian subcontinent still have nothing else to drink but meagre quantities of impure water, thus exposing themselves to infection.

The parasitic worm, 20-30 inches long, which causes dracunculiasis, migrates through the victim's body and eventually emerges causing intense pain, a blister and then an ulcer. The disease reappears each year during the agricultural season, handicapping farmers, mothers and schoolchildren already subject to harsh living conditions. Families affected by the disease experience great loss as their food stocks and savings dwindle. Gradually worn down by penury, these underprivileged people find themselves trapped in a vicious circle of poverty and disease.

Chagas disease affects 17 million people in 21 countries in Latin America and causes 45 000 deaths and 400 000 cases of heart and stomach disease annually. With WHO support, the six countries of the Southern Cone of the Americas – Argentina, Bolivia, Brazil, Chile, Paraguay and Uruguay – plan to eliminate the disease as a public health problem by the year 2000 using WHO-developed community-based insecticidal paints, fumigant canisters to destroy the insect vectors as well as detection boxes to verify the effectiveness of the control measures. Better diagnostic kits have been developed and blood screening improved. There is currently no effective drug for treatment of chronic infections, but two new products are on trial.

African trypanosomiasis (sleeping sickness) is transmitted by tsetse flies and is fatal if untreated. It kills an estimated 55 000 people a year, and sometimes erupts into widespread epidemics, as in Zaire in 1994.

WHO supported the application of the first new drug against the disease in 40 years – eflornithine – which is so effective it has been dubbed the "resurrection drug". However, treatment costs some $500 and is therefore beyond the reach of most affected countries without substantial subsidies.

Schistosomiasis (bilharziasis or snail fever), a water-related parasitic infection, affects 200 million people in 74 countries in the Americas, Africa and Asia and kills perhaps 200 000 people. Its effects include long-term, painful, swollen internal organs, anaemia, severe weakness and eventually permanent organ damage.

The disease mainly affects rural people engaged in agriculture or fishing. However, increased population movements have led to its introduction into a growing number of urban areas in northwest Brazil and Africa, and in refugee settlements. Similarly irrigation projects in many countries, in particular the building of dams, have resulted in an explosion of the snail population which harbours the parasites, and caused the disease to spread. Thus in addition to its toll of deaths, the disease hinders development and severely reduces the work capacity of many farmers and others.

Onchocerciasis has been brought under control in 11 countries through a massive WHO-administered programme against the blackfly vector.

Safe and effective drugs such as praziquantel are available, but their cost – although as little as $0.30 to treat one patient – prevents their widespread use which could allow control of the disease. At the request of Kenya, Malawi, Nigeria and Zambia, which together have more than 30 million infected people, WHO has succeeded in negotiating a reduction in the price of the drug with the manufacturers.

The potential population at risk of **leishmaniasis** is put at some 350 million and about 13 million people are infected. Transmitted by sandflies, the leishmaniases are a complex of parasitic diseases with a wide range of clinical symptoms. Visceral leishmaniasis, also known as kala-azar, is the most severe form and is nearly always fatal if untreated. It caused some 500 000 cases and more than 80 000 deaths in 1992. Cutaneous leishmaniasis, also known as oriental sore, causes some 1.5 million cases a year.

The disease is mostly rural, but is moving into a number of Latin American cities. Some 90% of the visceral cases occur in Bangladesh, India, Nepal and Sudan. Epidemics in India and Sudan in 1992 claimed most of the victims. About 90% of cutaneous cases occur in Afghanistan, Brazil, Islamic Republic of Iran, Peru, Saudi Arabia and Syria. Resistance is increasing so that cheaper, more easily administered drugs are needed.

Lymphatic **filariasis** is transmitted by mosquitos carrying the filarial parasite. It infects around 100 million people, 45 million of whom are in India. The disease leads to elephantiasis where the legs become grossly swollen and infected with sores, a debilitating condition with serious economic and social consequences, affecting many young working adults of both sexes. Patients are often shunned and isolated because of their disfigurement.

Drug therapy supplemented by vector control can be used to fight the disease. The main drug used for treatment is diethylcarbamazine (DEC) given once yearly, and costing around $0.10 per person. Part of the problem with con-

trol of the disease is that in many areas where it is endemic, it is not seen as a public health priority. China has seen a dramatic reduction in infection levels during the past decade. In India and Africa, which together account for 90% of all cases, there has been no decline in filariasis infection during the past 10 years and in several areas there has even been an increase.

WHO estimates that one-quarter of the world's population is subject to chronic **intestinal parasitic infections** which have insidious effects on growth, nutrition and cognitive function in children, and on the development of girls and women. Most of those affected live in developing countries. Ascaris causes clinical symptoms in as many as 214 million people, Trichuris in 133 million and hookworm in 96 million. Incidence of giardiasis is around 500 000 per year and prevalence of Entamoeba histolytica infection around 50 million.

Although mortality from intestinal parasites is low, the absolute number of deaths is fairly high because so many people are infected. It is estimated that in 1993 hookworm killed 90 000 people, Entamoeba histolytica 70 000 and Ascaris 60 000. The infections are spreading rapidly in slums, shanty towns and squatter settlements, a trend that is likely to continue with increasing and unplanned urbanization.

The consequences of manifestations of Ascaris, Trichuris and hookworm are promptly reversed by treatment with albendazole, levamisole, pyrantel and mebendazole. Mebendazole is produced at a substantially lower cost in generic form and is available at $0.027 per dose. Chemotherapy is part of a control strategy recommended by WHO which also includes health education and promotion of environmental health. Anthelminthics in single oral doses are also recommended for pregnant or lactating women.

Hepatitis B is the most deadly of the hepatitis group of virus diseases. It is a health concern particularly in Asia, sub-Saharan Africa and the Pacific basin. It is acquired from blood and body fluids of an infected person, usually through

WHO estimates that one-quarter of the world's population is subject to chronic intestinal parasitic infections which have insidious effects on growth, nutrition and cognitive function in children, and on the development of girls and women.

sex or sharing injecting drug needles. It can also be passed on from mother to baby. Apart from producing a severe and sometimes fatal liver condition, hepatitis B is a major cause of liver cancer.

At least 350 million people are chronic carriers of the virus. One-quarter will die of liver cancer or cirrhosis of the liver. There are some 4.2 million acute clinical cases each year, sometimes involving jaundice and death of the patient. Hepatitis B is estimated to have killed around 1 million people in 1993. Some 10 000 of these deaths were from fulminant hepatitis, around 663 000 from liver cancer and 344 000 from cirrhosis.

By the end of 1994, 73 countries had started routine vaccination of infants against hepatitis B. One of WHO's vaccination targets is that all countries should integrate hepatitis B vaccination into their national immunization schedules by 1997. Sadly there is little chance that the target will be met, because adding this vaccine is likely to cost another $1.50 on top of the $1 for conventional childhood immunizations. The additional annual cost, with administration and delivery overheads, would be some $200 million. The world is not willing to find the sum, albeit modest.

As pointed out in the section on adolescent health, **sexually transmitted diseases** (STDs) impose a huge health burden across the world. Some 236 million people are estimated to have trichomoniasis, with 94 million new cases a year. Chlamydial infections affect some 162 million people, with 97 million new cases annually. There are an estimated 32 million new cases of genital warts each year and 78 million new cases of gonorrhoea. Genital herpes infects 21 million people each year, and syphilis 19 million. More than 9 million people are infected each year with chancroid.

Many, if not all, STDs could be avoided if condoms were used. Most STDs can be treated effectively and cheaply, the cost of treating genital ulcer disease, for instance, being between $0.5 and $4 per person. But there are problems in the supply and accessibility of services, compounded by fear of stigma by patients and the attitude of some service providers.

HIV and **AIDS** continue to spread relentlessly. WHO estimates that in 1994 HIV prevalence among adults worldwide was over 13 million (*Map 6*). Male homosexuals are still at risk, but worldwide most adults with HIV infection are heterosexual men and women. The virus also affects people injecting drugs and, decreasingly, those receiving infected blood and blood products.

Some 6 000 people are becoming infected each day. In parts of Africa and Asia the spread of the virus seems remorseless. In southern and south-eastern Asia HIV infections were estimated at 2.5 million – a million more than in 1993.

In parts of northern Thailand 20% of 21-year old military recruits and 8% of women attending antenatal clinics are infected, yet HIV was virtually unknown in the country in 1987. In India infection rates have tripled since 1992. In China there has been a steep rise in the number of reported STDs, showing how vulnerable that huge country is to the spread of HIV. The HIV infection rate in Asia went from 12% of the global total in 1993 to 16% in 1994.

Infections are spreading in northern Africa and the Near East. In Latin America and the Caribbean there have been an estimated 2 million infections, with a rapid increase in Brazil. Some

Map 6. Estimated distribution of HIV-infected adults alive (including persons with AIDS), late 1994

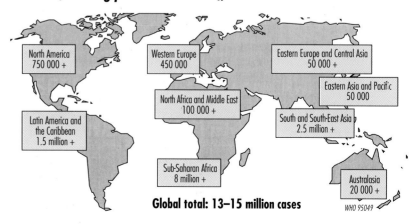

By the year 2000 the cumulative total of HIV infections worldwide could reach 30-40 million.

1.5 million infections have occurred in northern America, western Europe and Australia. There is concern at the growing number of infections in eastern Europe and central Asia, where economic crisis, unemployment, armed conflicts and major population movements could all favour the spread of the virus.

In sub-Saharan Africa, the part of the world worst affected, the estimated total now exceeds 10 million infections, with slightly more women infected than men. In 1980 HIV appears to have affected just a few areas of Africa with a prevalence of less than 0.1%; it now exceeds 10% in a few countries. One study in Botswana found that between 16% and 24% of sexually active females were HIV positive. Another in Nigeria among STD patients found a 22% HIV positive rate.

By the year 2000 the cumulative total of HIV infections worldwide could reach 30-40 million. In addition to new infections there will also be a huge increase in the number of AIDS cases. It is estimated that 4 million adults and children have developed AIDS since the start of the pandemic. The cumulative total is projected to reach nearly 10 million by the year 2000.

Because of the age group affected, AIDS is having an economic impact out of proportion to the numbers of people dying. It causes illness, disability and death among employees and their families. Worker productivity declines, firms have higher medical costs and they eventually lose staff with valuable training and skills. At the same time, as more of the population becomes ill and personal income drops, consumer markets shrink. Recent reports suggest AIDS has so affected agricultural productivity in some areas that increasing mechanization will be needed to maintain and harvest crops.

The disease is having a dramatic impact on the costs of health services. In many urban hospitals of central and eastern Africa 50% or more of medical ward beds are occupied by AIDS patients. In Zaire a single admission to Kinshasa's main hospital for a child with AIDS costs the equivalent of several months of an average salary. Altogether,

between 1992 and 2000, it is believed that the developing countries will be spending more than $1 billion on health care for AIDS patients.

In addition to their toll of death and bereavement and their vast economic burden, HIV and AIDS are inflicting untold damage in anxiety and worry.

In terms of prevention, condoms have been shown to make a difference. In Thailand STDs have fallen by 77% between 1986 and 1993. In Harare (Zimbabwe) STD rates decreased by 63% between 1990 and 1993 following condom promotion. In some groups reducing the number of sexual contacts and increasing the number of stable relationships have brought about a marked reduction in new infections. If sufficient effort is put into preventive work, encouraging changes in sexual behaviour can occur. AIDS, perhaps more so than any other disease, shows that behavioural scientists are as much needed as molecular biologists in the effort to slow the spread of the virus.

During the years 1979-1993 just over half the cases and 75% of the deaths from *plague* were in Africa. Three African countries registered plague in 1993 – Madagascar, Uganda and Zaire. Plague was also recorded in five Asian countries in 1993 – China, Kazakhstan, Mongolia, Myanmar and Viet Nam. Other cases were reported in Peru and the USA.

Plague is a disease of rodents and spreads from them to humans mainly by rat fleas biting first a sick rat and then a person, thus transmitting the bacillus of the disease, *Yersinia pestis*. Plague patients should be treated with antibiotic drugs such as streptomycin, kanamycin, chloramphenicol and tetracycline, which are effective provided they are used properly and in time.

The outbreak of plague in India in 1994 was a stern reminder to the world that a dreaded disease often regarded as a scourge of the past still exists. In 1993, 2 065 cases recorded in 10 countries, with 191 deaths, were notified to WHO. These figures were well above the annual averages (1 212 cases and 130 deaths) for the previous 10 years.

The Indian outbreak provoked unprecedented international concern about the disease, because of evidence that this was plague in its pneumonic form – which can be transmitted from person to person – rather than bubonic plague, which is more common but less infectious. This led a number of countries to impose restrictions on travel to and from India and many health authorities made provisions for quarantine measures. Among many other public health precautions, the Indian authorities introduced health checks for passengers departing on international flights.

In response to the outbreak, WHO issued travel advice based on the International Health Regulations, and set up an international team of experts which conducted a thorough investigation of the epidemic. The results suggested that a limited outbreak of pneumonic plague occurred in Surat, which many thousands of people had fled in panic, and involved far fewer cases than the number reported. No evidence was found of plague spreading outside Surat, and no imported, confirmed plague was detected in any other country.

Noncommunicable diseases

Diseases of the circulatory system killed an estimated 10 million people in 1993, or about 19% of the global total. In the developed world they claimed the lives of some 5.4 million people and were responsible for 47% of deaths. In the developing world they accounted for 4.2 million deaths, which although they constituted only 11% of all deaths in that part of the world, amounted to nearly as many as the number in the developed world.

In 1994 WHO published the world's biggest ever study on heart disease, covering 75 000 episodes in 1985-1987 among men and women aged 35-64. It found that the likelihood of heart attack was 12 times higher among men in North Karelia (Finland) than in Beijing (China), 9 times higher among women in Glasgow (United Kingdom) than women in Catalonia (Spain) and 7

times higher among women in Belfast (United Kingdom) than among the Spanish women. In terms of heart attacks per 100 000 population, the rates in males stood at 915 in North Karelia, 823 in Glasgow and 781 in Belfast. This compares to male rates of 240 in Toulouse (France), 187 in Catalonia and 76 in Beijing. Heart-attack rates per 100 000 for women were 256 in Glasgow and 197 in Belfast, compared to 37 in both Beijing and Toulouse, and 30 in Catalonia. While risk factors such as smoking, diet, blood pressure and cholesterol undoubtedly play a role, their differential effects in population groups require further research.

Findings from WHO's multinational monitoring project (MONICA) reinforced the evidence on differences between the sexes in terms of heart attacks – men aged 35-64 being 4 or 5 times more at risk than women of the same age.

Heart disease is commonly characterized as a lifestyle disease of the affluent, but there is also clear evidence that it is a problem in poor countries because of lifestyle changes. In addition rheumatic heart disease killed some 400 000 people in developing countries in 1993, even though it is easily preventable.

Rheumatic fever is caused by streptococcal bacteria and is spread in overcrowded highly contagious living conditions. In the case of repeated attacks of sore throat, severe damage to the heart valves may occur if the disease is left untreated. Five or more years of regular monthly treatment with penicillin at $1 per dose can prevent damage to the heart. This avoids heart-valve surgery at a cost of between $4 000 and $40 000 per patient.

Rheumatic heart disease strikes the young – those aged 5 to 35. WHO estimates that some 370 000 new cases of rheumatic fever and 150 000 recurrences take place each year, producing an annual toll of some 300 000 new cases of rheumatic heart disease. There are estimated to be at least 2 million children aged 5-15 with rheumatic heart disease in India alone.

Hypertension or high blood pressure is the most common cardiovascular dis-

The outbreak of plague in India in 1994 was a stern reminder to the world that a dreaded disease often regarded as a scourge of the past still exists.

order. Globally 8-18% of adults have high blood pressure, the normal value being defined as under 140/90 mmHg. This condition is a major contributor to heart disease as well as to stroke, kidney failure and other problems.

In the USA alone the condition affects an estimated 50 million people – or almost 1 in 4 adults; each year 29 million working days and $2 billion in earnings are lost to the country due to hypertension-related illnesses.

Lifestyle changes such as losing weight, reducing excessive salt and alcohol intake and increasing levels of physical activity can all help to lower blood pressure. Drugs such as diuretics and beta-blockers are widely prescribed for hypertension in industrialized countries but their cost can be prohibitive in the developing world.

Stroke and *other cerebrovascular diseases* killed about 4 million people in 1993, representing 7.5% of total global deaths from all causes. Stroke is a major cause of handicap in middle-aged and elderly people, causing partial paralysis or impairment to speech and other mental faculties. Stroke patients pose a growing problem in developed countries but their needs are largely ignored, with rehabilitation services given low or no priority. The care for such individuals falls largely on families.

Cancer killed some 6 million people in 1993. The majority of the deaths occurred in the developing world, although cancer is widely perceived to be a disease of industrialized nations. In the developed world there were around 2.5 million cancer deaths, contributing some 22% of the total. By contrast the 3.5 million cancer deaths in the developing world made up just 9% of the total. There were estimated to be some 20 million cancer sufferers in the world in 1994, with 9 million new cases a year. (*Box 7*).

An analysis carried out in 1993 by the International Agency for Research on Cancer (IARC) looked at worldwide cancer mortality trends in 24 geographical areas, using 1985 data. Worldwide, lung cancer was the biggest single killer in men, accounting for 22% of cancer deaths. In women breast cancer was the

main cause of cancer deaths in developed countries and the second cause in the developing world after cervical cancer. Another frequent cause of death for both sexes was stomach cancer, followed by liver cancer in men and colon cancer in women. The researchers estimated that 20% of all cancer deaths could be prevented if tobacco smoking was eliminated.

Deaths from cancer of the liver and of the cervix, both major problems in the developing world, could be substantially reduced by vaccination against hepatitis B and the introduction of cervical smear test programmes. If all countries were able to introduce an effective community-wide screening programme as in Finland, 76% of the world's deaths from cervical cancer – expected to reach around 276 000 by the year 2000 – could be prevented. A vaccination campaign against hepatitis B in countries with high rates of carriers could reduce deaths from liver cancer by at least one-half. Liver cancer is expected to kill some 296 000 men and around 137 000 women by the end of the century.

By the year 2000 there are expected to be about 4 million deaths annually from cancer in males worldwide, up from 3.1 million in 1990, and 3.2 million female cancer deaths (up from 2.6 million). Of the projected male cancers around 2.3 million will occur in the developing world and 1.6 million in the developed. Of the female cancers almost 2 million will occur in the developing world and about 1.2 million in the developed.

WHO estimates that in 25 years' time new cases of cancer each year (not deaths) in developed countries will have increased from roughly 4 million today to 5.5 million. In the developing world the figure will have doubled from 5 million to 10 million. Almost two-thirds of cancers over the next 25 years will occur in the developing world. Approximately 20 million people are alive with cancer at present; by 2015 there will probably be more than 30 million.

Chronic obstructive pulmonary diseases such as chronic bronchitis and emphysema killed nearly 2.9 million people in 1993, representing about 6%

Box 7.
Main cancer killers
(all countries, 1993)

Trachea, bronchus and lung	1 035 000
Stomach	734 000
Colon and rectum	468 000
Mouth and oropharynx	458 000
Liver	367 000
Female breast	358 000
Oesophagus	328 000
Cervix	235 000
Lymphoma	221 000
Pancreas	214 000
Leukaemia	207 000
Prostate	182 000
Bladder	135 000
Ovary	123 000
Uterus	64 000
Skin	37 000

of total deaths. The number of sufferers in the world is put at 600 million. This is the second largest known category of persons with a single disorder recorded by WHO. At the same time there are believed to be 275 million asthma sufferers in the world, although WHO has no data on the number of deaths each year due to this condition.

In the United Kingdom respiratory diseases account for one-quarter of general practitioner consultations. The most prevalent of them, chronic bronchitis, afflicts 8-17% of the population. These data are typical for Europe, but there are also widespread problems in developing countries. Data from four African countries show that 10-20% of adults have chronic bronchitis. Similar figures have been obtained from India and Nepal. Of the 2.9 million deaths from chronic obstructive lung diseases, nearly 2 million were in the developing world.

Indoor pollution from fuels like brown coal in China, or wood and cattle dung in Africa, is the main risk factor in the developing world whereas in developed countries it is cigarette smoking. There is increasing concern that air pollution and car exhaust emissions may be adding to the rising number of asthma cases.

Diabetes mellitus is a growing public health problem in both developed and developing countries. A recent WHO expert group estimated that more than 100 million people will suffer from diabetes by the end of this century – 85-90% of them with the non-insulin-dependent form (NIDDM). Older people and urban dwellers are more susceptible to NIDDM. In Europe the prevalence is 2-5% of the adult population. Recent surveys indicate a prevalence of diabetes in the Indian subcontinent of 10% rising to 25% by the age of 60. On the Pacific island of Nauru and among the Pima Indians of Arizona in the USA, half the population aged 30-64 are affected, and it is predicted that 1 in every 5 North Americans will develop the disease by the age of 70. NIDDM is strongly associated with the adoption of a Western lifestyle, with risk factors including obesity, lack of physical exercise

and inappropriate diet, and is thus potentially preventable.

Insulin-dependent diabetes mellitus, which usually starts in childhood, requires daily insulin injections and continual vigilance against taking too much or too little insulin. In developing countries the prohibitive cost of insulin can mean that the condition is a death sentence. Even in the best-controlled cases, with both forms of the illness, there is a greatly increased risk of heart disease, kidney failure, blindness and gangrene leading to limb amputations. These complications are extremely costly, both to the individual and to society. One recent estimate put the cost of diabetes in the USA alone, both direct and indirect, at $92 billion a year.

Congenital and *hereditary diseases* are growing public health concerns. 25-60 per 1 000 liveborn infants are estimated to have congenital abnormalities. Rapid progress in molecular genetics is making it increasingly possible to screen for inherited conditions, particularly single gene defects such as thalassaemia and cystic fibrosis, and is at the same time opening the way to their treatment.

Such techniques will alert parents to the possibility that their child will be badly handicapped, while having ethical and resource implications for health services and society as a whole. Couples face the moral dilemma of deciding whether or not to opt for an abortion in countries where this is permitted. In the case of diseases like Huntington chorea, where the effects will not become apparent until late middle age, there is a real question of whether people want the knowledge of what is going to happen to them.

Society has to decide how widely genetic screening services should be organized, and how much effort should be put into counselling couples about the implications of the tests. The dilemmas are likely to increase rapidly as new disease-causing genes are being discovered virtually every week. When genes are found that contribute to common illnesses such as heart disease, cancer and mental illness, the decision about whether to set up screening programmes

Diabetes mellitus is a growing public health problem. More than 100 million people will suffer from diabetes by the end of this century.

or not will become even more acute. There will probably be growing consumer pressure for such services and hard decisions will have to be made about what health resources should be devoted to them.

Mental health

Where in the global burden of disease should sorrow rank? Bereavement, separation, loss or betrayal can cruelly undermine the human spirit. The pain of emotional wounds may last a lifetime. The burdens of sorrow, depression and anxiety, the silent misery of loneliness and rejection, particularly amongst many elderly people, are largely ignored.

Mental ill-health is at the bottom of the medical pecking order. Only the most severe cases, such as schizophrenia or manic depression, receive what minimal care there is, even in developed countries. Moreover there are disturbing signs that society would sooner have such patients wandering the streets homeless than provide them with the care they need. The stigma of "madness" is still a potent barrier in preventing ill people from receiving help.

Some 500 million people are believed to suffer from neurotic, stress-related and somatoform disorders (psychological problems which present themselves as physical complaints). A further 200 million suffer from mood disorders, such as chronic and manic depression. Mental retardation affects some 83 million people, epilepsy 30 million, dementia 22 million and schizophrenia 16 million. In developed countries a huge proportion of visits to family doctors are not for medical, but for social or emotional reasons. The problems are to do with low income, unemployment, poor housing and failed relationships, and in most cases it is beyond the doctor's power to help.

Safeguarding mental health in increasingly fractured societies, where many of the previous cultural and social support systems (such as the family or organized religion) are weakening, is an awesome challenge reaching far beyond the realms of health care systems.

On average smoking kills 6 people a minute. Smoking is already killing 3 million people a year worldwide.

Smoking

Smoking is emerging as the world's largest single preventable cause of illness and death. WHO estimates that there are about 1.1 billion smokers in the world today. About 300 million (200 million males and 100 million females) are in the developed world – but in developing countries there are nearly 3 times as many, some 800 million, almost all males. Globally 30% of adults (48% of men and 12% of women) are regular smokers. On average smoking kills 6 people a minute. Smoking is already killing 3 million people a year worldwide. If current trends continue, this figure is expected to reach 10 million by 2020.

In the USA, where traumatic deaths are more common than in other developed countries, the risk from smoking still far outweighs other dangers. On average among 1 000 20-year olds who smoke cigarettes regularly, about 6 will die from homicide; about 12 will die in motor-vehicle accidents; about 250 will be killed by smoking in middle age; and a further 250 will die from smoking in old age.

A recent British study concluded that smoking can kill or cause harm in 24 different ways. The diseases include cancers of the lung, mouth, pharynx, larynx, oesophagus, stomach, intestine, pancreas and bladder, leukaemia, chronic bronchitis and emphysema, pulmonary heart disease, tuberculosis, pneumonia, raised blood pressure, heart disease, blocking of the arteries, brain clots, two forms of brain haemorrhage, sudden rupture of the aorta, stomach ulcers and duodenal ulcers. There are additional dangers for women. Smoking can cause ectopic pregnancies, increase the chances of a premature or underweight baby, and contribute to cervical cancer by damaging the lining of the cervix.

Many studies, including the above, have highlighted the benefits of stopping smoking, even after many years. Those who stop at any age before serious disease sets in have mortality rates in later life considerably lower than those who continue. It's never too late to stop.

Oral health

Oral health status, as reflected by the average number of decayed, missing and filled teeth among 12- year old children, is generally improving in the developed world; the developing and the least developed countries, however, showed a deterioration. Globally there were about 1.9 billion persons with dental caries; 165 million with periodontal diseases; and 13 million with edentulism. The number of teeth still possessed by elderly people is a crucial factor in whether they can eat properly and hence affects their quality of life, yet oral health is given low priority in many countries.

Inadequate access to basic or emergency oral health care is now better recognized to be a problem in the developing world. Although reliance continues to be placed on dentists and the use of expensive, sophisticated equipment, the situation is now that affordable and sustainable activities are being identified to extend care to rural and disadvantaged urban communities.

Accidents, violence and suicide

External causes of mortality, such as motor-vehicle accidents, fires, homicide and violence, suicide and occupational disease and injuries killed some 4 million people in 1993, or nearly 8% of the global total (of which some 3.1 million were in the developing world). Falls, fires, drowning and such like killed 1.8 million people. Motor and other road accidents killed 885 000 people and there are estimated to be about 10 million such accidents each year. Around 779 000 people took their own lives and some 302 000 died as the result of violence or homicide. Occupational accidents claimed the lives of 220 000 people. These figures do not include those killed in wars and civil unrest.

Poverty, as in almost every other category of illness and disease, plays a significant role in increasing the chances of death and injury from external causes. Unsafe working conditions, inadequate housing, poor road engineering, the widespread use of agricultural and other chemicals without proper precautions, social breakdown and even military conflict are all rooted in economic and social factors.

Injuries remain in most countries a persistent, and in some cases increasing, cause of death and disability, particularly among the young. Accidental injury is an important cause of death in children and young adults (5-29 years). If homicide is added, external injury is a leading cause of mortality in this age group. There are an estimated 330 000 occupational injuries every day in addition to a daily toll of about 600 deaths. Almost 70 million new cases of occupational disease result each year from various exposures at work. Agrochemicals cause around 3 million poisonings annually, mostly among poorly-protected labourers in the developing world. Despite the scale of the problem, up to 90% of workers have no access to occupational health services.

Blindness and deafness

There were about 38 million blind people worldwide in 1990, with an increase of 10 million since 1978. Some 58%, or 22 million people, are aged 60 and above. In addition there are estimated to be a further 110 million people with impaired vision. Based on population trends, there may be 54 million blind people over the age of 60 by the year 2020, of whom more than 50 million will be in developing countries. It has been estimated that 42 million people worldwide suffer from moderate to serious hearing loss. However, this is likely to be a gross underestimate.

Women's health

In developed countries in 1991 there were more than 200 000 deaths of women aged 15-44, of which 4 000 were ascribed to maternal causes. In the developing world there were almost 2.4 million deaths among women in the same age group; and of those, more than 500 000 – almost one-fifth – were ascribed to maternal causes, most of which are easily preventable. Chief among the

There are an estimated 330 000 occupational injuries every day in addition to a daily toll of about 600 deaths.

causes were haemorrhage, sepsis, hypertensive disorders of pregnancy and obstructed labour. Each year millions of children are left without mothers, thus imperilling their own immediate safety and leaving them vulnerable to psychological and social burdens in the future.

Box 8. *The mother-baby package*

The mother-baby package is based on the following principles considered to be the four pillars of safe motherhood:

(1) to ensure that individuals and couples have the necessary family planning information and services to plan and space pregnancies;

(2) to provide proper antenatal care so that complications of pregnancy are detected as early as possible and correctly treated;

(3) to give all birth attendants the necessary knowledge, skills and equipment to perform a clean and safe delivery and provide postpartum care to the mother and baby;

(4) to make essential obstetric care available for all high-risk cases and emergencies.

The package recommends a basic set of simple interventions focused on the main causes of maternal mortality:

■ before and during pregnancy: information and services for family planning; STD/HIV prevention and management; antenatal registration, checkups; treatment of existing conditions (e.g. malaria, hookworm); advice regarding nutrition and diet; recognition, early detection and management of complications such as eclampsia, bleeding, abortion and anaemia; tetanus toxoid immunization; iron/folate supplementation;

■ during pregnancy: clean and safe delivery; access to essential care at a health centre or hospital for bleeding, eclampsia, prolonged/obstructed labour and other complications;

■ after delivery (mother): prevention and early detection of postpartum haemorrhage, sepsis and eclampsia; postpartum care including support for breast-feeding, family planning and STD/HIV prevention services, tetanus toxoid immunization;

■ after delivery (newborn): resuscitation when necessary; keeping the baby warm; early and exclusive breastfeeding; prevention, early detection and treatment of infections including ophthalmia neonatorum and cord infections.

If properly applied the mother-baby package could avert about 270 000 maternal deaths or over 50% of the estimated total of around 500 000 per year, as follows:

Cause of death	Percentage of deaths averted
Haemorrhage	55
Sepsis	75
Eclampsia	65
Obstructed labour	80
Unsafe abortion	75
Indirect causes	20

The differences in maternal mortality between countries are unacceptable. In Europe maternal mortality is 50 per 100 000 live births. In Africa the figure is more than 670 – a 13.5 times greater risk. Maternal mortality in the 47 least developed countries is appallingly high, reaching more than 700 per 100 000 live births in 1991.

Of the half a million estimated maternal deaths in 1991, haemorrhage caused about 130 000, with an estimated 14 million cases annually. Indirect causes during pregnancy, such as anaemia and malaria, resulted in 100 000 deaths out of a total of some 13.5 million cases. Sepsis took the lives of 75 000 women, with around 12 million cases. Obstructed labour was responsible for the deaths of 38 000 women, with some 7 million cases. Hypertensive disorders of pregnancy, including pre-eclampsia and eclampsia, took the lives of about 60 000 women, with an estimated 7.1 million cases a year. Between them haemorrhage, sepsis, abortion, hypertensive disorders and obstructed labour are believed to have resulted in the long-term or permanent disablement of some 18 million women (from conditions including severe vaginal, urinary and bowel problems, ectopic pregnancies and infertility).

There were an estimated 140 unsafe abortions for every 1 000 live births in 1990. Among 1 000 women aged 15-49 there was one unsafe abortion in market-economy countries, 23 in countries in economic transition, 16 in developing countries, and 28 in the least developed countries. In all, there are around 20 million such procedures each year, causing the death of almost 70 000 women.

Globally it is estimated that in 1990 more than half the number of pregnant women were anaemic, a threat not only to the mother's health, but also a contributing factor to low birth weight. Hookworm infection due to *Necator americanus* and *Ancylostoma duodenale* exacts a heavy toll especially on women of childbearing age and young girls, causing iron deficiency anaemia which is associated with high maternal mortality and morbidity and lowered school performance. WHO has estimated that 44 million pregnant women worldwide are infected.

While there are justifiable concerns over the lack of medical care for pregnant women in developing countries, there are complaints in many developed countries that the process of birth has become overmedicalized, so that a natural human process has been turned into an illness. The widely differing rates for Caesarean deliveries, for instance, suggest that birth practices are influenced by factors other than strictly medical indications. In the Americas, Caesarean section accounted for 5% to 34% of deliveries.

Over the past three decades contraceptive use has increased by 27% globally, rising in the less developed world from 9% in 1960-65 to 53% in 1990. But there are still very large unmet family planning needs. In order to meet United Nations goals to reduce world population growth, contraceptive rates in developing countries will have to increase to 59% by the year 2000.

In summary 72% of maternal deaths are due to the same five main causes around the world: haemorrhage, sepsis, obstructed labour, eclampsia, and unsafe abortion (Box 8). The remaining 28% are due to conditions aggravated by pregnancy, such as malaria or hepatitis. In the wider sense, however, it is poverty and lack of knowledge which cause these deaths. Underlying the medical causes of death are the social, economic and cultural determinants of poor maternal health. Low levels of resources and skills and insufficient infrastructure make access to care difficult. In addition, women's inferior socioeconomic status, lack of resources and decision-making power and low levels of education hinder their use of appropriate maternal health care services. Premature death and suffering related to childbearing are not inherent in the human condition – they are rooted in the social, cultural and economic settings of the countries where they are prevalent. Something can be done about them.

Health of the elderly
A greying world

The increase in the number of old people in the world will be one of the most profound forces affecting health and social services in the next century. In the poorest countries childhood deaths are a key factor in average life expectancy. But for people who do survive, increasing numbers will go on to old age.

Overall the world's population has been growing at an annual rate of 1.7% during the period 1990-1995 – but the population over 65 years is increasing by some 2.7% annually. Of a world total of 355 million people over 65 in 1993, more than 200 million were in the developing world, where they made up 4.6% of the population, and more than 150 million in developed countries, where the proportion was 12.6%.

The process of population aging started earlier in Europe, and 18 of the 20 countries with the highest percentages of elderly are in that region (the others are Japan and the USA) where 13-18% of the population is already over 65 years.

However, the most rapid changes are being seen in the developing world, with predicted increases in some countries of up to 400% among people aged over 65

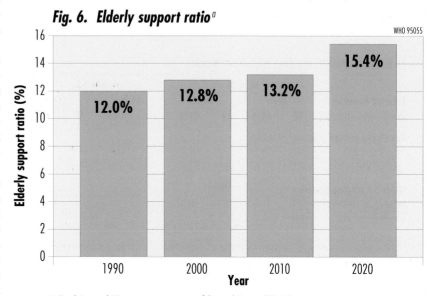

Fig. 6. Elderly support ratio[a]

WHO 95055

(bars: 1990 = 12.0%, 2000 = 12.8%, 2010 = 13.2%, 2020 = 15.4%; y-axis: Elderly support ratio (%); x-axis: Year)

[a] Population aged 65 or more as a percentage of the population aged 20–64.

Box 9. Healthy life expectancy

More than 15 years ago all the countries of the world resolved that their health and health-related activities should have a common goal of ensuring by the year 2000 that the health status of all people should be such that they can at least work productively and participate actively in the social life of their community. Recent studies, however, indicate that mortality reductions have sometimes resulted in a lengthening of life in unhealthy circumstances, increased inactivity and dependency as well as higher rates of chronic, non-lethal impairments, particularly among the elderly. It is being asked whether people are surviving chronic diseases only to live on in poor health.

Since life expectancy measures are of limited interest when it comes to assessing the quality of years lived, whether during early years or at higher ages, several other measures are being investigated – for example disability-free life expectancy, quality-adjusted life expectancy, disability-adjusted life years (used by the World Bank), and years of productive life lost (used by OECD). More recently the notion of "health expectancy" has emerged, referring to life expectancy in a given state of health, as governed by a broad range of positive and negative factors such as impairment, disability, handicap and self-rated health.

Although international comparisons are not yet possible due to differences in study design, data collection and the classification of health expectancy, recent research has shown the following patterns of general life expectancy (LE) and disability-free life expectancy (DFLE) in different groups of countries.[a]

Independent life expectancy[b]

Selected countries	At birth				At age 65			
	Male		Female		Male		Female	
(latest available data)	LE	DFLE	LE	DFLE	LE	DFLE	LE	DFLE
Developed market-economy countries								
Canada, 1986	...	...	...	...	14.9	8.1	19.2	9.4
Finland, 1986	...	...	...	...	13.4	2.5	17.4	2.4
United Kingdom, 1991	...	...	...	...	14.3	13.6	18.1	16.9
Least developed countries								
Myanmar, 1989	...	...	...	...	12.0	11.1	13.5	12.8
Other developing countries								
Egypt, 1989	...	...	...	...	12.1	10.8	13.3	10.1
Fiji, 1984	...	...	...	...	13.1	10.5	14.6	10.4
Malaysia, 1984	...	...	...	...	13.4	11.9	15.0	12.7
Republic of Korea, 1984	...	...	...	...	12.9	9.0	15.0	9.4
Sri Lanka, 1989	...	...	...	...	13.2	12.3	14.7	13.4
Tunisia, 1989	...	...	...	...	12.7	11.3	13.8	11.4

Functional limitations-free life expectancy[c]

Selected countries	At birth				At age 65			
	Male		Female		Male		Female	
(latest available data)	LE	DFLE	LE	DFLE	LE	DFLE	LE	DFLE
Developed market-economy countries								
Australia, 1992	74.5	58.2	80.4	64.0	15.4	6.4	19.2	9.0
Spain, 1986	73.2	61.6	79.6	63.6	15.0	7.0	18.4	6.9
Other developing countries								
Indonesia, 1976-1977	51.8	47.8	54.8	50.3	...	...	...	...

[a] Based on figures prepared by the Network on Health Expectancy and the Disability Process (REVES), which brings together researchers in this field.

[b] Refers to the average number of years an individual is expected to live without restrictions in a number of basic activities of daily living such as getting in and out of bed, dressing and washing, and "instrumental" difficulties such as cooking, shopping and housekeeping, if current patterns of mortality and difficulties in performance of the activities continue to apply.

[c] Refers to the average number of years an individual is expected to live free of limitations on functions such as bending, picking up objects and walking, if current patterns of mortality and difficulties in performance of the functions continue to apply.

during the next 30 years. In developed countries the increase will in some cases be as low as 30%.

Alongside an increase in the number of people aged over 65 there will be a dramatic rise in the numbers of "old old" – people over 80. In 1993 they constituted 22% of those over 65 in the developed world and 12% in the developing world.

Longer life – or more years of sickness?

The world elderly support ratio (the number of people over 65 years compared to those aged 20-64) in 1990 was 12 elderly to every 100 people of working age (*Fig. 6*). It is estimated that the figure will be 12.8 in the year 2000 and 13.2 in 2010. The estimated ratios for 1990 and the year 2000 were 20 per 100 and 23 per 100 respectively in developed countries and about 9 per 100 and 10 per 100 in the developing world. In other words while population growth during 1990-2000 is estimated to be 17%, the increase in the number of elderly is likely to be 30%.

Over the coming decades there will be more old people depending on fewer people of working age as the source of funding for their health care. Advances in health technology extend life, but do not necessarily improve the quality of life and raise profound ethical questions. Unless the productivity of the working age population increases, there will be a growing problem of providing the funds to enable the elderly to live a secure and dignified life.

One of the most difficult questions facing health planners and politicians trying to allocate funds, as well as the community and individuals themselves, is whether increased life expectancy means more health or simply more years of sickness. Life expectancy is not an indicator of the burden of disease in old age. Increasing age makes self-reliance more difficult. It brings growing disability, an inability to walk, climb stairs or carry heavy loads and so on. In addition old age can bring financial hardship and poverty, as even well-provided pensions – where they exist – are less than people earned when they were working.

Surveys of elderly people in many countries show a high prevalence of such conditions as arthritis and rheumatism, deafness and poor vision and of specific chronic diseases of the heart, brain and lungs including stroke, dementia and cancer. Old people are therefore high consumers of health services. In some countries the elderly comprise just 10% of the population but use 30% of the services. One of the most urgent but so far generally neglected needs with regard to care of the elderly is to find some sort of measure to assess disability and the quality of life, in order to provide information for setting of service priorities, planning and evaluation (*Box 9*).

Dementia and arthritis

Two of the most cruel burdens facing the elderly are dementia, particularly Alzheimer disease, and the crippling pain of rheumatism and arthritis. Both can destroy quality of life, place huge burdens on relatives and carers and take up immense amounts of health and social service resources, although neither is amenable to cure.

Dementia, a sad and often lengthy life in limbo for both sufferers and their relatives, is believed to affect at least 22 million people worldwide. The chances of contracting the condition increase with old age so that those over 80 have a 15-20% chance of becoming demented. In the 12 states that comprised the European Union in 1994 it was estimated that in 1990 there were some 3.5 million people with dementia. By 2000 this figure is expected to increase to about 4 million.

Joint pain caused by rheumatism and arthritis places a huge burden on the elderly, but it largely goes unrecorded and is sometimes seen by doctors as the inevitable price of getting old which patients have to bear. However, it is the reason for massive prescriptions of pain-killers, which in themselves can go on to cause stomach ulcers, and is the prime reason for the lengthening queues of elderly people needing hip replacement and other joint-replacement operations. The prevalence of rheumatoid arthritis in different populations has been estimated at 1-5%. Assuming an average prevalence of 3%, this suggests that there are at least 165 million people in the world with rheumatoid arthritis.

The second most prevalent chronic rheumatic disease is osteoarthritis, which can strike all the joints. It causes significant damage to the knees in about 20-40% of people over 70 years and to the hips in 5-10% of those aged over 65.

Another significant skeletal disease in the elderly, particularly among women, is osteoporosis – thin bone disease. Around 1 in 3 women aged over 50 are affected and are thus far more prone to bone fractures, including broken hips and damage to the vertebrae. About 1.7 million hip fractures occurred in 1990 throughout the world. Global data on vertebral fractures and forearm fractures are not available.

Institutional care

Long-term care of the frail elderly is becoming one of the most hotly-debated medical and political issues in many developed countries, and the developing world too will soon have to wrestle with it.

The question of who pays for the care of the elderly will increasingly confront health services around the world, and society as a whole. Old age can bring great loneliness. In developed countries, and increasingly in developing ones, a woman whose husband dies in his 60s may still have 20 or even 30 years of life as a widow. If people are not to be left destitute, and uncared for at the end of their lives, more attention must be given to social mechanisms for the support of the elderly and the means to fund them. The problem of aging need not be medicalized. Making the aging population a resource for the community and health services enables them to live in dignity.

> *Dementia, a sad and often lengthy life in limbo for both sufferers and their relatives, is believed to affect at least 22 million people worldwide.*

General health issues

A changing world

In the last 10 years there has been an unforeseen and overwhelming global trend towards the democratization of political systems, accompanied by much greater participation of people in determining their own future. On the other hand, while the end of the cold war has relieved the tension between East and West, regional and local conflicts and warfare have persisted and emerged. Hopes were high for reduced spending on arms and greater spending on health development. So far this "peace dividend" has not materialized, or has been absorbed by peace-keeping efforts, leaving meagre resources for human development. At the same time the growth in the numbers of refugees and displaced people in recent years due to these conflicts has raised serious problems for the provision of health care, and it would be naive to expect that they will disappear.

The changing demographic picture across the world together with the rapid shift towards urbanization will have profound implications for the delivery of health services. The unplanned and often chaotic growth of megacities in the developing world will pose particular challenges, as poor sanitation and housing will encourage the spread of infectious diseases.

Long-term growth in the capacity of the world economy to supply goods and services has led to widespread improvements in material standards of living for most of the world's population. Nevertheless, although the gap between developed and developing countries has narrowed, the gap between the developing and least developed countries has widened. Although it is difficult to see such a situation changing markedly over the next five years, efforts to bridge the gap must be a priority for the world community.

Poverty has continued and will continue to be a major obstacle to health development. Poverty is perhaps the major single determinant of individual, family and community health. The number of poor people has increased substantially, both in the developing world and among underprivileged groups and communities within developed as well as developing countries – particularly in the slums of the great cities. During the second half of the 1980s, the number of people in the world living in extreme poverty increased, and was estimated at over 1.1 billion in 1990 – more than one-fifth of humanity. An expanding world population and a growing elderly population carry with them the danger of an even greater divide between those who are rich and those who are poor. Here again is a formidable gap to be bridged.

Against any optimism about the global economy throughout the remainder of this century and beyond should be set a number of major uncertainties. There has been a disproportionate flow of resources from the developing to the developed world – poor countries paying money to rich countries – because of debt servicing and repayment and as a consequence of prices for raw materials that favour the latter at the expense of the former. Structural adjustment policies aimed at improving economic performance of poor countries have in many cases made the situation worse. The words of Robert McNamara, spoken in 1980 when he was President of the World Bank, still hold true: "The pursuit of growth and financial readjustment without a reasonable concern for equity is ultimately socially destabilizing".

A worrying trend is growing unemployment, especially in developing countries without social security arrangements to cushion those out of work. Studies in a number of countries have documented the severe negative effects of unemployment on health. Long-term unemployment is creating a new class of "untouchables" – by excluding a large group of people from the mainstream of development and society. This is yet another gap to be bridged. The unemployed are a potent reminder of the dangers of assuming that the general prosperity of a county will trickle down to all its members. Even in the

> *Poverty has continued and will continue to be a major obstacle to health development.*

wealthiest countries, such as the USA, the gap between the richest and the poorest has widened dramatically over the past decade, with a fall in real wages for the poorest. In many countries of the former USSR the transition to market economies has been accompanied by a drastic fall in real wages for many. The inability to buy nutritious food or secure warm and dry accommodation is producing a legacy of ill-health which may persist for many years until the benefits of market economies become tangible for all.

There is considerable concern about the adverse health effects of continuing environmental degradation, pollution and the uncontrolled dumping of chemical wastes, diminishing natural resources, depletion of the ozone layer and predicted global climatic changes. The Rio Declaration which emerged from the 1992 United Nations Conference on Environment and Development, with its action plan on sustainable development, gives hope that action will be taken to protect the future health of the people of the world by preventing environmental disaster.

The global situation with regard to literacy is improving, but this improvement is not shared equally. Illiteracy, common among women and the poor, continues to impede health and social development. Overall adult literacy is expected to increase to about 80% by the end of this century, although for the least developed countries a rate of only about 50% is projected. Millions of young people still have no opportunity for education, and girls and women continue to be underrepresented in the classroom; female literacy remains a key developmental issue.

The structure of the family, the basic unit of support and nurture for both children and adults, is undergoing rapid evolution in many parts of the world. Extended networks of relatives are being lost and traditional patterns of social support thereby weakened.

A growing number of women in the developed as well as in the developing world are entering paid labour for economic reasons. This produces welcome household resources but can also increase social strains within families and place even greater burdens on women. However, because of the cultural and social setting, aging populations function as resources in the family, community and health services in most developing countries.

Changing social mores, with a move towards shorter marriages and more divorces in many countries, are leading to family breakdowns which have repercussions for individuals and for social services that may be called in to provide help for children and single parents. Family breakdown has an impact on the behaviour of young people with regard to sexual relationships and the use of tobacco, alcohol and other drugs. The ultimate family breakdown involves the situation where children leave home or are pushed out, and are forced to eke out an existence on the streets. The millions of street children across the world pose a severe challenge to health and welfare services. It is difficult to prescribe easy remedies as to how these children should be reached and their future looks bleak unless there is a major societal shift in accepting that their care should have priority.

The soaring world population will strain to the limit the ability of social, political, environmental and health infrastructures to cope. It more than doubled from 2.5 billion in 1950 to almost 5.6 billion in 1993, with 4.4 billion in the developing world, including 556 million in the least developed countries.

In many least developed countries geographical, climatic and environmental factors remain a major factor of ill-health. Many have wet tropical climates which favour mosquitos and other vectors of disease. Many still lack safe water and sanitation, upon which the control of many infectious diseases largely depends. In 1990, more than 1 billion people in the developing world lacked access to safe drinking-water.

The soaring world population will strain to the limit the ability of social, political, environmental and health infrastructures to cope.

Sustaining health for all

The concept of health for all has changed the world's thinking about how health should be provided. Placing equity of access to health at the heart of health-care delivery and giving greater emphasis to achieving this goal through primary health care has become a global blueprint. However, sustaining both the belief in the concept and its practical implementation has been difficult, partly because of the economic recession, cost implications, resistance to change and political problems in diverting resources from other areas towards health. The fundamental reason is that there is still little recognition at the political and policy levels of the close interrelationship between poverty and ill-health. It is disheartening to see that resources are allocated for high technology medicine while ignoring the basic human needs of the poor. A rectification of this imbalance will not only make the poor more healthy but also less poor. There is a need for strong and sustained leadership to continue to push forward the goals of health for all – and there is an overwhelming need to retain and implement the principle of fair and equal treatment for all, so ensuring better health and not merely improving access to health care.

Environmental health hazards

Acute and chronic exposures to chemicals during their production, storage, transport and use affect many millions of people every year. Agrochemicals alone lead to about 3 million poisonings a year. Millions more people are exposed to toxic chemicals in food, drinking-water or air.

Naturally occurring toxic chemicals are of particular concern in poor communities with a traditional lifestyle, especially if people get most of their food and all their drinking-water from local sources. Geochemical conditions may create particularly high concentrations of trace elements in food or water, leading to local endemic diseases, which may affect millions of individuals.

Epidemics of poisoning in such circumstances have occurred in India and Afghanistan and are major concerns in other parts of Asia and in Africa. The extent of the health impact is unknown, but more is being learned about local situations as national chemical safety programmes are formulated.

Resources for health

Resource constraints are forcing most countries to reassess their existing arrangements for health care financing and provision. Many countries are concerned about responding to growing demand and rising costs in the health sector, while ensuring value for money. They are under pressure to develop health policies and structures that provide better quality health care while using resources more efficiently. Governments are experimenting with alternative forms of health financing (Box 10). In many countries a complex mix of funding sources and care providers in both public and private sectors is emerging. The role of government is increasingly being seen to create an enabling environment in which all providers are regulated, monitored and evaluated in a coordinated fashion. But there is unease in some quarters that governments may be silently withdrawing from their responsibilities to provide care, acting instead as ring masters while other actors do the work.

In many countries the skills mix of health teams is still inappropriate, and personnel are poorly distributed. Market forces alone cannot achieve a rational and cost-effective mix. Scientific and technical developments, changes in health care delivery and the need to keep costs from rising all mean that innovative thinking is required about how health professionals are to be deployed. This will probably require radical departures from traditional roles.

> *In many countries the skills mix of health teams is still inappropriate, and personnel are poorly distributed. Market forces alone cannot achieve a rational and cost-effective mix.*

Health infrastructure

The most protective vaccines, the most effective drugs, the most powerful antibiotics – none are of use if the people in need do not get them. Although the concepts of the rational use of drugs and the essential drugs list are widely accepted, the lack of foreign currency for purchasing needed supplies inhibits countries' ability to provide primary health care to a great many people. About 1 billion people worldwide do not have regular access to local health services.

At the same time cheap, effective, life-saving treatments sit unused on shelves while people are dying because still in many areas of the world the delivery systems to get them to the population do not exist or are inadequate. Health infrastructure – the buildings and equipment, the staff, the drugs and vehicles – is central to good health. Health infrastructure is the skeleton which supports health care (including the specialist care given in hospitals) and without which no health programme can be sustained.

Increasingly there is a recognition that health services must be provided close to the people who need them – and an integrated, cost-effective approach is necessary. People need a point of entry – the first level of care – which not only provides a basic package of services appropriate to the epidemiological situation but also facilitates access to all other services which may be needed.

Although in the past special programmes for specific diseases – immunization for example – have produced truly impressive results, it is no longer sustainable or cost-effective to set up self-contained taskforces for individual illnesses. Fragmented and duplicated health care services jeopardize the effective use of available health resources, and the continuity and sustainability of services. It makes no sense for doctors and nurses to vaccinate children if at the same time children die because they do not have antibiotics against pneumonia or oral rehydration therapy for diarrhoea.

It makes no sense for child health nurses to give superb care to infants but ignore the fact that a mother has ma-

---

Box 10. Health systems on the move

Most countries today are attempting to adopt health policies and structures that provide better care, use resources more efficiently and encourage appropriate health-seeking and health-promoting behaviour.

The poorer countries increasingly recognize that health and socioeconomic development cannot be pursued independently, and that limited resources have often been spent mainly on large urban hospitals as a result of poor investment decisions taken in a context of underdeveloped planning, budgeting and financial information. However, systems that are well organized and geared to making health care accessible to all nevertheless require considerable resources. User charges, community-financing and health insurance have all been envisaged as funding mechanisms.

The richer countries are struggling to maintain or improve standards while controlling total health spending which has been spiralling owing to aging populations, the introduction of expensive technologies and rising expectations. Concerns from the patient's point of view have been waiting lists, impersonal attention and limited freedom in the choice of health care provider. Organizational change, healthy lifestyles and the environment are high on all agendas.

Two important concerns are shared by most countries. The first is to redefine the roles of the key actors – governments, care providers, consumers and health financing agencies. The second, common to many low- and middle-income countries, is to find new financing mechanisms that will generate additional resources and bring greater efficiency and equity in health. The financing and provision of care is increasingly seen as a partnership between government and other actors.

In countries changing from a centralized-controlled to a liberal economy, health care has deteriorated and health policies are in a state of flux, as financing shifts from integrated public models to more pluralistic systems. Reform in such circumstances focuses on improving the quality and effectiveness of services, and lays more stress on the private sector.

Governments are seeking to reduce bureaucracies, and the role of ministries of health is shifting from direct delivery of care towards monitoring and regulation. Unfortunately, many ministries lack the structural and managerial capacity as well as the political strength to implement the necessary reorientation. Many are in fact starting to decentralize services to the district level, hoping this will lead to improved management, efficiency, accountability and responsiveness. The private sector is being given a greater role through such mechanisms as selling or otherwise disposing of public assets and making lump-sum subsidies, seconded personnel, tax-free equipment and bonus incentives available to nonprofit health care providers. Within this framework the public system is encouraged to compete for patients through policies which combine payment on a contract basis with free choice of provider by the patient. Thus government resources are tied to the consumer not to the facility. User fees are structured in such a way as to encourage patients to make effective use of health services.

Insurance is another way of financing health care. Social health insurance is generally compulsory, the premiums being paid by both the employer and the employee. Beneficiaries are principally those in formal employment. Private health insurance is normally voluntary and premiums reflect the level of risk of the insured individual. Community-based insurance schemes also cover the self-employed and those who are not in formal employment. They tend to be voluntary and some problems arise in enrolling poor people.

laria. It makes no sense to provide effective family planning but let people remain ill and contagious because they fail to complete their tuberculosis medication. Integration is the key to effective delivery of care.

There cannot be high-technology hospitals in every part of every country and there does not need to be. Instead, a tier system should be created, with established links between the various levels of the health services, with the peripheral health units seeing the majority of cases and feeding through to district-level hospitals, which in turn can refer patients to more specialized centres if need be.

It is also important for the infrastructure to provide health promotion and disease prevention as integral parts of the services, rather than only concentrating on curative medicine.

It is only when services are integrated, and the duplication of staff and equipment eliminated, that the costs of health care delivery can be seen for what they are – excellent value for money. With good infrastructure it is possible to demonstrate that lives can be saved in many cases for a few cents.

Essential drugs and pharmaceuticals

Half the world's population still lacks regular access to the most needed essential drugs. Poorly coordinated drug policies and strategies, inefficient procurement, inequity in distribution, inadequate assurance of quality, unaffordable prices and inappropriate use are commonplace.

Drug promotional practices and a lack of objective therapeutic information continue to cause concern especially in developing countries, many of which do not yet have a national drug policy and the necessary capability to deal with these problems. Meanwhile in many countries the demand for drugs is growing while resources decrease. Without access to essential drugs, health care systems cannot function. Developing countries in particular need international support in assuring drug and vaccine quality.

Traditional medicine

Traditional medicine continues to be an important part of health care in many developing countries, and various "alternative" or complementary therapies enjoy a widespread following in developed countries. Traditional medicine has not, however, been incorporated into most national health systems, and the potential of services provided by traditional practitioners is far from being fully utilized. There is a continuing need for better assessment of the benefits of alternative forms of medicine including traditional ones.

Rationing of health care

When expectations rise and sophisticated technology is available but money is short, what treatments should be rationed? If there has to be a choice between who lives and who dies, how is it to be made? An experiment in Oregon (USA) of trying to draw up a list of essential treatments and a list of treatments that would not be offered was criticized as being a mechanistic approach to health care. The World Bank's *World development report 1993* on investing in health proposes that in poor countries there should be no complex heart surgery, no treatment other than pain relief for cancer, no provision of expensive drugs for HIV/AIDS and no intensive care for severely premature babies. This proposal was criticized as applying a balance-sheet mentality to health care. But the question of setting priorities and the need for rationing will not go away. With an aging population and advancing medical technology it is only a matter of time before this issue, with all its ethical implications, comes to the fore (*Box 11*).

Least developed countries and debt relief

The 47 countries which are designated as least developed share similar burdens – hostile environments, endemic diseases, poverty and huge debts. They have inadequate access to whatever health services are available, the lowest

Half the world's population still lacks regular access to the most needed essential drugs.

levels of literacy and the highest rates of sickness and death (*Table* 6). But no country can provide adequate health services without resources to pay for them. Total donor aid to the least developed countries was estimated at around $17 billion a year in 1991. Their collective debts amounted to some $114 billion, and annual repayments were around $4.4 billion. Without debt relief the burdens on them will certainly increase, as will the misery of many millions of their citizens.

Conclusions

The problems outlined in this report are of awesome magnitude, but they are not insoluble. As Helen Keller said, "Although the world is full of suffering, it is also full of the overcoming of it". The potential exists; what is needed is a universal awareness of the problems and the collective will to solve them.

It is not inevitable that millions of children should die of preventable diseases, or that hundreds of millions of

---

Box 11. *From medical ethics to social ethics*

Since antiquity, the doctor/patient relationship has been governed by systems of medical ethics drawn from the Hippocratic, Chinese, Indian and other traditions. All held that the patient's good transcended other considerations. The physician determined what was the patient's good. Modern codes have added a social dimension, a responsibility for the health – the good – of society and humanity in general, and a concern for justice. Health for all, with its emphasis on social justice, on the equitable allocation of resources and on the responsibility of communities and individuals for their own health, is an expression of this change, and thus represents an ethical as well as a social goal.

The transformation of medical ethics has been stimulated partly by the progress of medical biotechnology and partly by profound social changes, associated with a recognition of human rights and freedoms, and of individual autonomy. Many medical choices can no longer be made purely on the basis of medical science. The emphasis on the social good has confronted lay individuals, whether policy-makers or patients, with ethical decisions and choices, requiring them to share with or often replace the physician or the scientist in determining what is ethically acceptable and good, to balance the patient's interests with those of society.

The explosion of expensive medical technologies, often of limited value to the patient, and the rise in people's expectations, have accentuated the problem of making the best use of limited resources. Policy-makers must set priorities to guide the allocation of resources among health goals and between health and other social goals. They do so under many pressures – social, economic, political, technological and ethical. They are forced to make choices with often tragic consequences. In principle medicine can use the full potential of modern biotechnology – for transplanting organs, for assisting reproduction, for postponing death, for reducing hereditary diseases, even for manipulating the genetic make-up of human beings. In practice the policy-maker, by controlling resources and trying to reflect the dominant values of society, determines how much medicine can do, and even which patients

may benefit. Thus the good of society and individual good may come into conflict.

For their part individual patients today exercise autonomy and informed consent in deciding whether or not to accept or continue with treatment, even to continue to live, to become a subject of research, to permit the use of personal health data for study purposes, to be told – or not told – the truth, to permit the use of embryos, to donate organs and to withdraw life-support systems.

Individuals, like communities, are often the subjects of research, such as trials of drugs or vaccines or epidemiological studies. Some living in deprivation or even oppression are liable to exploitation. Researchers have a particular ethical responsibility to safeguard the rights of such people and to observe scrupulously the ethical principles of beneficence, avoidance of harm, and justice. WHO has mechanisms for assuring the ethical soundness of research with which it is associated, and seeks at the same time to strengthen national capacities for addressing ethical issues relating to health policy and research. WHO's main partner in this respect is the Council for International Organizations of Medical Sciences. Together the two bodies have over the years convened a series of conferences on health policy, ethics and human values, and prepared ethical guidelines for biomedical and epidemiological research.

Health for all, a new and universal concept, has exerted a profound influence on health development during the last decades of this century. Equity is now seen as the major policy and ethical requirement in organizing, financing and managing health care systems. Although approaches to ethics necessarily differ, since they depend on evolving cultural patterns, social beliefs, forms of community organization and religious convictions, WHO is endeavouring to elaborate certain universal principles. In this respect the Organization's role is not to rule on what is right or wrong, but to promote dialogue between different schools of thought and to strive for consensus.

Table 6. Comparative data for selected high-income countries, severely indebted low-income countries in 1991, and other least developed countries

WHO Member States (ranked by GNP per capita)	Population (000) 1993	Life expectancy at birth 1993	Infant mortality rate 1993	Under-5 mortality rate 1992	Physicians 1989-1991		Nurses 1989-1991		Health expenditure per capita (US$) 1990	GNP per capita (US$) 1992[a]	Adult literacy rate (both sexes) 1990	Adult literacy rate (female) 1990
					Number	Rate per 100 000 population	Number	Rate per 100 000 population				
High-income countries												
Japan	124 959	79	5	6	204 690	164	...	...	1 538	28 190	...	...
United States of America	257 840	76	8	10	606 680	238	...	...	2 765	23 240	...	...
France	57 379	77	7	9	169 051	300	...	...	1 869	22 260	...	...
Low-income/severely indebted countries (excluding least developed countries)												
Ghana	16 446	56	80	170	628	4	3 998	27	15	450	60	51
Nigeria	119 328	53	95	191	17 954	17	64 503	61	10	320	51	40
Kenya	26 090	59	65	74	1 063	5	2 692	11	16	310	69	59
Low-income/severely indebted countries (least developed countries)												
Mauritania	2 206	48	116	206	127	6	886	44	18	530	36	27
Liberia	2 845	55	126	217	...	...	...	...	14	(460)	40	29
Zambia	8 885	45	82	202	...	...	...	...	17	(450)	73	65
Mali	10 137	46	158	220	...	...	...	...	15	310	32	24
Niger	8 529	47	123	320	142	2	2 036	26	16	280	28	17
Madagascar	13 259	56	110	168	1 392	12	3 124	26	7	230	80	73
Zaire	41 166	51	93	188	2 496	7	27 601	74	5	(230)	72	61
Guinea-Bissau	1 028	44	139	239	...	...	...	...	16	220	37	24
Burundi	5 995	48	105	179	317	6	...	...	30	210	50	40
Uganda	19 246	43	101	185	704	4	2 332	14	8	170	48	35
Sierra Leone	4 494	43	142	249	...	...	...	...	4	160	21	11
Somalia	9 517	47	121	211	...	...	...	...	8	(120)	24	14
United Republic of Tanzania	28 783	51	100	176	...	...	...	...	4	110	...	...
Sudan	27 407	52	98	166	...	...	...	...	34		27	12
Myanmar	44 613	58	81	113	3 242	8	...	...	...	...	81	72
Other least developed countries												
Botswana	1 352	61	60	58	...	...	...	...	139	2 790	74	65
Vanuatu	161	...	...	...	15	10	...	...	67	1 210	...	...
Samoa	158	...	...	...	50	32	...	...	20	940	...	...
Cape Verde	395	68	42	...	...	...	...	...	64	850	67	...
Solomon Islands	354	70	27	...	52	16	447	140	117	710	...	...
Kiribati	75	...	...	...	14	20	116	163	...	700	...	...
Lesotho	1 882	61	78	156	74	4	874	50	28	590	...	...
Yemen	12 977	53	105	177	2 640	23	6 480	55	20	(520)	...	...
Comoros	607	56	88	...	57	10	155	29	28	510	...	...
Guinea	6 306	45	133	230	773	13	...	...	17	510	24	13
Maldives	234	64	54	...	15	7	...	...	...	500	...	...
Benin	5 075	46	85	147	323	7	1 384	31	19	410	23	16
Central African Republic	3 258	47	104	179	113	4	259	9	18	410	38	25
Togo	3 885	55	85	137	319	9	1 187	33	18	390	43	31
Haiti	6 893	57	86	133	...	...	...	...	27	(380)	53	47
Gambia	932	45	131	...	...	...	...	...	22	370	27	16
Sao Tome and Principe	127	...	...	...	61	51	233	196	38	360	...	...
Equatorial Guinea	379	48	116	...	99	28	154	44	28	330	50	37
Burkina Faso	9 788	48	116	150	252	3	909	10	7	300	18	9
Lao People's Democratic Republic	4 605	51	96	145	945	22	...	...	5	250	...	...
Rwanda	7 789	47	109	222	272	4	835	12	10	250	50	37
Bangladesh	122 210	53	107	127	...	...	...	...	7	220	35	22
Chad	6 010	48	121	209	147	3	86	2	12	220	30	18
Malawi	10 694	45	140	226	186	2	284	3	11	210	...	...
Cambodia	8 997	51	115	184	...	...	...	...	...	(200)	35	22
Bhutan	1 650	49	125	201	141	9	233	15	10	180	38	25
Nepal	21 086	54	98	128	1 124	6	601	3	7	170	26	13
Ethiopia	48 791 [b]	...	...	208	...	...	...	...	4 [c]	110 [c]	...	...
Mozambique	15 322	47	143	287	388	3	2 847	20	5	60	33	21
Tuvalu	13	...	...	...	...	...	...	...	...	...	...	...
Afghanistan	20 547	44	161	257	2 233	13	1 451	9	...	...	29	14
Djibouti	481	49	111	...	...	...	...	...	...	...	...	...

Source: Berthlemy JC, Lourc'h A. *Debt-relief and growth*. Paris, OECD Development Centre, 1994.

[a] Figures in brackets reflect the most recent estimate for the period 1987-1992.

[b] Excludes Eritrea.

[c] Includes Eritrea.

... Data not available or not applicable.

Box 12.   *New and re-emerging infectious diseases*

Some infectious diseases such as malaria, once thought to be on the verge of elimination as a public health problem, remain leading causes of death worldwide. The incidence of some has increased within the past two decades, and others pose a growing threat. A number are caused by hitherto unknown agents, such as hantavirus pulmonary syndrome.

Notable among the new and re-emerging diseases are infection by *Escherichia coli* 0157:H7, which has provoked foodborne outbreaks of severe bloody diarrhoea and kidney failure in several countries; multidrug-resistant pneumococcal pneumonia, which particularly affects children; cholera caused both by classical strains and by new biotypes — as recently illustrated among Rwandan refugees; dengue and the more severe dengue haemorrhagic fever, a life-threatening disease endemic in many parts of Asia and increasingly common in the Americas; and cryptosporidiosis, a waterborne cause of diarrhoea that affected over 400 000 people in a single outbreak in the USA in 1993.

Many factors, or combinations of factors, can contribute to disease emergence. New infectious diseases may result from the evolution of existing organisms; known diseases may spread to new geographical areas or new populations; or previously unrecognized ones may appear in persons living or working in areas undergoing ecological changes such as deforestation or reforestation, which make them more exposed to insect, animal or environmental sources of infection. Re-emergence of infectious diseases may result from the development of antimicrobial resistance in existing agents (e.g. gonorrhoea, malaria, pneumococcal disease) or a breakdown in public health measures against previously controlled infections (e.g. cholera, tuberculosis, pertussis).

Other causes include changes in lifestyle, particularly in overcrowded cities where population growth has outpaced supplies of clean water and adequate housing; the dramatic growth of international travel, which allows a person to be infected in one country and become ill in another distant corner of the world; and changes in food handling and processing which mean that foodstuffs may have originated thousands of miles away or have been prepared from many different animals.

To confront this challenge WHO seeks to strengthen global surveillance of infectious diseases; build international infrastructure to recognize, report and respond to new disease threats; create an applied research programme focusing on practical problems and realistic solutions; and reinforce prevention and control through targeted interventions.

Current WHO activities include regional and local projects on urban mosquito control to reduce the risk of dengue and yellow fever; research to develop new or improved vaccines for emerging diseases, and better methods of administering the products already available; collaborative projects and provision of grants to strengthen reference laboratories and WHO collaborating centres, which are the first lines of defence; and provision of training for technology transfer.

people should not have access to safe water or sanitation. Why, at the close of the 20th century, should huge numbers of women still be dying in childbirth? Why do we allow even greater numbers of children to become brain-damaged because of a lack of iodine in their salt, or to go blind because of a lack of vitamin A?

Although this assessment of global health status has been limited by a scarcity of epidemiological and other data, certain conclusions can be reached based on the most reliable information at our disposal.

The most powerful image that emerges is of widening gaps in health between the haves and the have-nots. Gaps not just between rich and poor, but between the poor and the poorest of all. Gaps not just between regions and countries, but between populations within those countries. There is a neglected underclass not just in every country, but in virtually every city. They are the street children, the unemployed, the elderly and the marginalized – including millions of women whose greatest disadvantage is their gender. There are also flagrant gaps in access to health care, between taking sophisticated national health services for granted and dying for want of a midwife.

The widening gaps in health status and in access to health care among countries and population groups far outdistance the gains made in global health improvements, and threaten the sustainment of those gains.

Globally life expectancy at birth has increased to about 65 years while mortality among infants and children under age 5 has fallen to about 62 and 87 per 1 000 live births respectively. However, the increase in life expectancy has been gained at a price: the extra years are accompanied by pain and a loss of dignity. Any comfort that can be derived from longer life expectancy must be tempered by the knowledge that about 6% of deaths in the world each year are still among children less than one week old.

At least 45 countries, with a total population of 850 million or about 15% of the world population, have not yet reached the minimum targets of life expectancy at birth of at least 60 years, and of mortality among infants and children under age 5 of below 50 and 70 per 1 000 live births respectively (see *Annex 3, Table A*).

The 80% immunization coverage in 1990 of infants against vaccine-preventable diseases is falling, possibly due to financial constraints in procurement of vaccines. Yet immunization, at a cost of roughly $10 per child, has protected more than 100 million infants over a 10-year period, and saved more than 20 million lives at a cost of about $1 billion. How much really is a billion dollars? About the same, in fact, as is spent on beer every 12 days in the USA, and by Europeans on cigarettes every 5 days.

Infectious and parasitic diseases are the leading causes of death worldwide. As campaigns for the global eradication of poliomyelitis, measles and neonatal tetanus move forward, and leprosy nears elimination as a public health problem, the major challenge is to enable those suffering from these diseases to be economically and socially productive. Similarly drug resistance will pose a challenge in the control of malaria and tuberculosis.

Alongside the pandemic of HIV/AIDS, the world is witnessing a re-emergence of diseases such as cholera, dengue haemorrhagic fever and plague (*Box 12*). Developing countries are bent low under a double burden of ill-health: while still struggling against major communicable diseases, they are having to contend with an expansion of noncommunicable diseases such as cancer and cardiovascular diseases as well as a surfeit of accidents and violence.

An aging population as well as rapid urbanization, particularly when accompanied by growth of urban slums, will be a driving force in future health development. Greater demands on land, with a depletion of natural resources, and on the working population – due to elderly dependency – are casting a worrying shadow, in respect not only of health but also of social development generally.

Although the global economy and agricultural production, particularly related to cereals, are growing faster than the population – a trend that is likely to continue – it is not the least developed countries that are benefiting; in fact they are being left behind.

The link between population, development, environment and health is so strong that health policy is no longer confined to the conventional health sector; more and more it is influencing – and being influenced by – social policy and ethical concerns.

The momentum generated by the global strategy for health for all by the year 2000 in ensuring more equitable access to health and health care has to be sustained and accelerated in a changing world. There is a need to shift emphasis from preventing death to preventing ill-health and enhancing quality of life. Allowing individuals to achieve their full health potential enables them to be economically and socially productive.

There is a need to shift emphasis from preventing death to preventing ill-health and enhancing quality of life.

Chapter 2
WHO's contributions to world health

Introduction

Chapter 1 showed that for most of the world's population every step in life, from infancy to old age, is taken under the twin shadows of poverty and inequity, with health care providers facing enormous problems in fighting disease and ensuring equal access to care – in other words in bridging the gaps in global health. The review also showed that people's health status can be improved, albeit gradually. The present chapter provides an overview of the many activities undertaken by WHO – in 1994 alone – to support countries in the improvement of health care. They range from the establishment of international norms and standards for biological substances, vaccines and pharmaceuticals to direct support in health emergencies. WHO's activities are governed broadly by its constitution that sets the attainment by all peoples of the highest possible level of health as the ultimate objective of the Organization and its Member States. WHO is a goal-oriented organization working to meet clearly defined objectives. These and related plans of action are determined by general programmes of work outlining for each six-year period a global health policy framework as well as a framework for WHO's action (the current eighth programme covers the period 1990-1995). Other detailed guidance is provided by four interrelated policy orientations agreed for WHO's work during the current 1994-1995 biennium: integrating health and human development in public policies; ensuring equitable access to health services; promoting and protecting health; and preventing and controlling specific health problems. At the same time pri-

orities have been set for each programme in the light of the results expected from WHO's two main functions of technical cooperation with countries and coordination of international health work. These are complementary and together include: advocacy of measures to improve health; stimulating and mobilizing specific health action and disseminating information; developing norms and standards, plans and policies; training; research promotion; direct technical consultation; and resource mobilization. The full extent of WHO's work cannot be fully reflected in this report, but examples are given of the different types of action. Regional highlights are also presented.

Child health[e]

WHO's work helps to save the lives of several million children every year. Through its global strategy for health for all by the year 2000, WHO promotes a coherent, integrated approach to all aspects of child care including childbirth. It gives priority to achieving the 1992 World Summit for Children target of reducing, by the year 2000, mortality in children under age 5 to a maximum of 70 per 1 000 live births through:

immunization of at least 90% of women and children aged under 1 year against childhood target diseases (diphtheria, pertussis, tetanus, measles, poliomyelitis, tuberculosis) eradication of poliomyelitis by the year 2000
reduction of measles cases by 90% and measles deaths by 95% by the year 1995
elimination of neonatal tetanus by the year 1995

> WHO's work helps to save the lives of several million children every year.

[e] The age groupings used for the purpose of this report are: children, including infants (under 5 years); school-age children and adolescents (5-19 years); adults (20-64 years); and the elderly (65 years or more). Where information cannot be assigned to one of these categories, it is given under *General health issues*.

- reduction in the annual number of cases of diarrhoea incidence by 25% and diarrhoea deaths by 50% in children under age 5
- a one-third reduction in mortality from acute respiratory infections in children under age 5
- virtual elimination of vitamin A deficiency and its consequences including blindness
- reduction in the number of children with low birth weight.

WHO estimates that *immunization* saved approximately 3 million people from dying from measles, neonatal tetanus, pertussis and poliomyelitis in 1993. However, some 2.1 million deaths still occur annually from the first three diseases as well as 114 000 cases of poliomyelitis. In a number of countries yellow fever and hepatitis B vaccine were added to the immunization schedule. In response to worldwide concern over injection practices, autodestruct syringes became more widely used for immunizations. The multivaccine jet injector that allows vaccines from different vials to be combined at the time of injection is at an early stage of development, while testing of time-temperature indicators for immunization was completed. In Africa a follow-up study of children immunized against hepatitis B was carried out in connection with research on the role of the virus in liver cancer.

The 1995 goal of *neonatal tetanus* elimination has already been attained by many countries and will ultimately be reached by many more – but only if routine immunization coverage is sustained and action in high-risk districts accelerated. In an effort to make the best use of limited resources WHO has given priority to countries that account for 80% of total cases and have an estimated mortality of 5 or more per 1 000 live births.

In response to the *diphtheria* epidemic in the Russian Federation and Ukraine, WHO worked closely with Member States to assure prompt investigation and reporting. A plan of action for diphtheria control in the European region was completed. Guidelines for case investigation, treatment of suspect

cases and laboratory testing were prepared. WHO has also worked with donors to ensure that necessary supplies of vaccines, antitoxin and antibiotics are made available. A European task force on diphtheria control was set up at the WHO Regional Office in Copenhagen, in order to accelerate progress in controlling the epidemic in eastern Europe and to reduce the danger of its spread.

In 1993 progress towards the *poliomyelitis* eradication goal was heartening. No cases were reported from the western hemisphere. In the Americas eradication has been pursued through a concerted effort by national governments and a consortium of donor agencies. Countries in Africa and the Eastern Mediterranean are now recording zero or low incidence. Globally, however, the steady decline in incidence from 1988 did not continue in 1992, when the reported rate rose by 6% compared with the previous year, primarily owing to an increase in South-East Asia. Efforts are being made to develop a more heat-stable poliovirus vaccine that can be delivered with a less rigorously maintained cold chain. Large donations for poliomyelitis eradication were coordinated with Rotary International, the United States Centers for Disease Control and Prevention, USAID, AIDAB and JICA.

Measles immunization coverage reached a peak of 80% in 1990; since then it has declined slightly and is currently only 78%. This has largely been due to a falling-off in international interest and support following achievement of the 1990 target of 80% immunization of children under 1 year, and disruption to services as a result of war and civil strife. The number of reported cases has continued to decrease. The goal of reducing measles mortality by 95% can be reached by 1995; but the goal of reducing incidence by 90% in every community will not be achieved.

In 1994 the region of the Americas committed itself to eliminating measles by the year 2000. Country after country has embarked on a campaign to interrupt transmission of the disease, and incidence is now at the lowest level ever. If the momentum is sustained the

The 1995 goal of neonatal tetanus elimination has already been attained by many countries and will ultimately be reached by many more.

Americas may well lead the way towards global elimination of this major killer of children.

WHO encourages self-reliance of countries in conducting immunization through basic health services. It cooperates with UNICEF in its initiative of supplying over 100 countries with vaccine worth over $65 million a year, representing 40% of the total global production. Major priorities are to at least sustain the accomplishments of previous years and to continue to strive for achievement of the 1992 World Summit for Children goal of immunization against the six vaccine-preventable diseases.

Recent years have seen increasing demands for WHO support for national programmes to control *diarrhoeal diseases* in children. By the end of 1994 virtually all developing countries had implemented plans of action. Nearly 42% of health staff in the countries had been trained in supervisory skills using training materials developed by WHO, and almost 30% of doctors and other health workers had been trained in diarrhoea case management, many of them in the more than 420 diarrhoea training units established in over 90 countries. It is estimated that nearly 85% of the population of the countries had access to oral rehydration salts at the end of 1994. Surveys indicated that 88% of mothers were aware of the need for continued feeding for children with diarrhoea and 77% of the need for increased fluids.

In close coordination with UNICEF, WHO has developed an integrated clinical approach to managing the main diseases of children: acute respiratory infections, diarrhoea, measles, malaria and other febrile conditions, malnutrition and anaemia. Within WHO, 10 programmes and units are participating in this initiative. The different guidelines in this field have been consolidated into four treatment charts. A training course on use of the charts was developed and pretested in Ethiopia, and a revised version will be field-tested in the course of 1995.

The last few years have seen a fairly rapid increase in the proportion of children having access to standard case management for *acute respiratory infections*, particularly pneumonia. By the end of 1994, 59 of the 88 target countries with high infant mortality rates had operational control programmes, and activities were in progress in districts where over 25% of children are at risk. WHO supports countries in formulating policies, planning programmes, implementing training and communications strategies and conducting evaluation surveys.

Particular emphasis is given to training in the management of acute respiratory infections. WHO supports courses for workers in first-level health facilities and referral hospitals on standard case management and distributes training and technical materials. Minimum requirements for monitoring the quality of training were established. More than 190 000 health managers, doctors, nurses and community health workers in over 60 countries have been trained so far.

WHO is involved in numerous studies on acute respiratory infections in Africa, Asia and Latin America. These include research on pneumonia in infants, including the effects of indoor air pollution; studies on the safety and efficacy of vitamin A supplementation in young infants to prevent diarrhoea and pneumonia; and field or clinical trials of vaccines against cholera, dysentery and respiratory infections. Other studies deal with the effectiveness of various antibiotic drugs in the treatment of acute respiratory infections in infants and malnourished children.

Technical and financial support for *nutrition* activities was provided to 62 countries, mostly in collaboration with FAO and UNICEF. A global database on child growth was established, and indicators and procedures for monitoring the prevalence of iodine, iron and vitamin A deficiencies were published in cooperation with UNICEF. WHO also issued a major report describing the effects of poverty on nutrition, on the basis of a collaborative study with the International Food Policy Research Institute (USA).

WHO cooperates with UNICEF in its initiative of supplying over 100 countries with vaccine worth over $65 million a year.

About 200 million children under age 5 are affected by protein-energy malnutrition; and some 36% of children in the developing world are underweight. Since 1993 WHO's efforts to improve infant and young child nutrition have focused on promoting breast-feeding. It has been calculated that breast-feeding could prevent the deaths of at least 1 million children a year. A new "baby-friendly hospital initiative", created and promoted by WHO and UNICEF, has proved highly successful in encouraging proper infant feeding practices, starting at birth. In Africa alone, where problems of infant malnutrition are especially acute, two-thirds of the countries have already implemented this simple, yet effective concept. Continued technical and financial support will be made available to more than 90 countries to give effect to the International Code of Marketing of Breast-Milk Substitutes. A workshop on supplementary feeding for children was held for African and Eastern Mediterranean countries.

In South-East Asia WHO collaborates with governments in establishing national nutrition policies and strategies and implementing programmes, with emphasis on common nutritional deficiency disorders. A South-East Asian regional nutrition network was set up and should lead to improved weaning, anaemia control and prevention of vitamin A deficiency and to the creation of national expertise in behavioural research. Iodization of salt to control iodine deficiency disorders has been promoted in Africa since 1987. Many countries now have a formal policy for this measure and seven have reached the objective of universal iodization.

Health of school-age children and adolescents

Increasing attention is being paid to the health of adolescents throughout the world in recognition of the impact of a rapidly changing world on their behaviour and the importance of this period of life in setting patterns which have lifelong implications. WHO supports activities focusing on adolescents in the areas of nutrition, mental health, sexuality and reproductive health including equity between the sexes, non-communicable and communicable diseases, health education, injury prevention and use of tobacco, alcohol and other drugs.

A joint UNICEF/WHO/UNFPA policy statement on the reproductive health of adolescents has been disseminated. WHO supported the formulation of adolescent health policies in more than 20 countries, and cooperated closely with many NGOs in promoting adolescent health. In 20 countries projects on street children were implemented jointly with the International Organization of Good Templars. Training and other materials were developed and widely distributed in collaboration with USAID, UNESCO, the Sasakawa Foundation and the Commonwealth Youth Programme. In South-East Asia adolescent health programmes are being carried out in Indonesia, Myanmar and Sri Lanka.

A regional plan of action on health and violence for the Americas has been formulated, which enshrines the principles of comprehensiveness, equity, political commitment, civic culture and knowledge as a basis for action and community participation. It seeks to prevent violence, diminish its effects on vulnerable groups and set up adequate care for victims.

WHO is re-evaluating the role of HIV/AIDS counselling and supports research on male-female relations in four countries, on risk-related sexual behaviour among young people in seven countries, and on household and community responses to HIV/AIDS in five countries. Member States in Africa are given technical support on preventing HIV infection in young people through health education, behaviour counselling, promotion of condom use and encouragement of a healthy lifestyle. Governments are being urged to include education on HIV/AIDS and sexually transmitted diseases in the school curriculum, and WHO worked with the

Breast-feeding could prevent the deaths of at least 1 million children a year.

Young People's Christian Association and IFRC on peer education projects on HIV/AIDS among out-of-school youth in three countries.

A multicentre study was started in three countries to explore areas of conflict between adolescents and adults which undermine healthy behaviour. A number of studies were supported in such fields as the capacity of health services to respond to adolescents' needs, the impact of deworming on the nutritional status of schoolchildren and comparisons of the effectiveness of albendazole and mebendazole in reducing intestinal wormload. Materials were produced in such areas as training of health professionals in adolescent health, and health facts for youth.

Health of adults

WHO activities focus on enabling the adult population to be economically and socially productive by reducing premature morbidity and mortality and enhancing their health potential. Health issues that are of particular relevance to adults include workers' health; human reproduction; tuberculosis; HIV/AIDS and sexually transmitted diseases; cardiovascular diseases; cancer; mental and neurological disorders; hereditary diseases; and alcohol and drug use.

Efforts are made to improve national capabilities to design and promote healthy work environments. A WHO global strategy on *occupational health* for all was formulated, an advisory body on workers' health was established, and recommendations were made for the reorientation of occupational health services in the new independent states. Guidelines and monographs are being produced on occupational respiratory diseases induced by organic dust and sensitizing agents, occupational exposure to selected metals, solvents and pesticides, and the carcinogenic risk to humans of various exposures. Since 1976 WHO has evaluated the health risks posed by exposure to close to 200 industrial chemicals and other substances.

Communicable diseases

In face of the mounting threat of **tuberculosis** WHO is seeking to mobilize major support from the public and private sectors, and a special account for tuberculosis was established within the Organization's Voluntary Fund for Health Promotion. Programmes were reorganized in a number of countries, and projects launched with financial support from the World Bank and ODA. Standardized short-course chemotherapy for tuberculosis is starting to be introduced in most countries of South-East Asia according to WHO guidelines. In India, a revised national plan was drawn up which will accord higher priority and greater resources to tuberculosis control, including financing by the World Bank. A similar outcome is expected from reviews carried out in Indonesia and Nepal. WHO is the implementing agency for tuberculosis and leprosy control under the World Bank's fourth population and health project in Bangladesh.

Research activities have produced some important results which might have profound implications for policy. A study of rifapentine suggests that it is a promising new drug. Another new drug, sparfloxacin, whose initial assessment in tuberculosis control was supported by WHO, will be tested in a large trial of multidrug-resistant tuberculosis. Epidemiological studies have demonstrated the important interaction between HIV and tuberculosis. A study in Uganda of the feasibility of tuberculosis chemoprophylaxis for HIV-infected persons suggests that this intervention is not easily transferable on a large scale in a developing country setting. A study in India, partly funded by ODA, is assessing ways of involving private practitioners more effectively in tuberculosis control.

First medium-term plans were formulated for 129 national **HIV/AIDS** programmes, and second-generation plans for 70. Sexually transmitted diseases and HIV/AIDS programmes have been integrated in most African countries, some 80 developing countries are

WHO has evaluated the health risks posed by exposure to close to 200 industrial chemicals and other substances.

National programmes for the prevention of coronary heart disease have been introduced in 41 countries.

supported in the implementation of sentinel HIV surveillance, and a new bulk purchase agreement for HIV test kits for developing countries was concluded. Approximately 60 million condoms were ordered for developing countries at reduced unit cost. Senior managers and other staff from 80 countries were trained in HIV/AIDS programme management, and distance learning material on blood safety for blood transfusion service staff was published. High priority was given to AIDS prevention in South-East Asia, where national AIDS committees were established, education and information of health workers and the general population started, and laboratory facilities strengthened for screening of blood for HIV.

A WHO-endorsed phase I (safety) trial of an HIV candidate vaccine took place for the first time in a developing country. WHO has characterized HIV strains in about 80 blood specimens from evaluation sites and made them available to scientists and manufacturers. Vaccine testing sites were strengthened in four developing countries. An epidemiological model of mature sexually transmitted HIV epidemics in central and eastern Africa is being validated, and a major research project in western Africa including prostitutes and their clients supported. A method for evaluating the effectiveness of HIV prevention was developed in collaboration with USAID and distributed worldwide.

Guidance on HIV testing is being issued, and a policy developed on restrictions for HIV-positive travellers including migrants and refugees. During the Rwanda emergency guidelines were disseminated on reducing HIV transmission in emergency situations, including a list of essential supplies for blood transfusion. Support is being given to several countries to develop a comprehensive blood safety policy in order to reduce blood transmission of various infections including HIV/AIDS. WHO works in partnership with hundreds of NGOs and networks of organizations in this field. Intensive work is under way with other

United Nations bodies to ensure a smooth transition towards the new joint and cosponsored programme.

Noncommunicable diseases

WHO is establishing a network of centres and a database in support of a global programme to monitor and prevent **cardiovascular diseases**, and continued to coordinate the 10-year, 26-country MONICA project which monitors trends and determinants in cardiovascular diseases and measures the effectiveness of interventions. The first comparable rates of incidence and case fatality for heart attacks were published. National programmes for the prevention of coronary heart disease were introduced in 41 countries. Cardiovascular disease risk factor trends over five years were evaluated, and a cardiovascular and alimentary comparison study was carried out in 20 countries. Guidelines for coronary heart disease and hypertension control are being prepared.

Noncommunicable diseases have a number of common risk factors and an integrated approach to their prevention is promoted. Sixteen INTERHEALTH demonstration projects have been set up worldwide (9 of them in developing countries) to assess the effectiveness of integrated community-based intervention. The related CINDI programme now covers 21 countries in Europe.

WHO prepared a manual on palliative care for home care givers and guidelines on **cancer** pain relief, updated a model list of 24 essential drugs for cancer chemotherapy and produced a handbook and policy documents on the public health approach to combating cancer. National cancer control programmes are being developed in over 40 countries that have established "foundation measures" which provide at low cost the essential managerial, political, educational and legislative framework for the implementation of effective national measures. An epidemiological study on diet and cancer is under way. Support was given for the implementation of national cancer pain relief and palliative care policies in over 46 countries, and an active international network of national experts, collaborating centres and NGOs has been established. The appropriate use of relatively simple therapies, especially radiotherapy, is promoted, as is education on palliative care and the use of opioids. A study was completed on the role of human papillomaviruses in cervical cancer.

The applicability of modern technology to the control of **hereditary diseases** is being investigated. An international multicentre study was launched on the predictive value of individual genetic and environmental risk factors for hereditary hypercholesterolaemia. Guidelines were issued on monitoring for birth defects and for the control of haemoglobin disorders. A European register of patients with cystic fibrosis and an Asia/Pacific working group on the control of haemoglobinopathies were established. As part of efforts to strengthen national genetic programmes, WHO supported a number of international studies, including the international human genome research project, and cooperated with the World Federation of Hemophilia in studying modern treatment methods emphasizing gene therapy.

With regard to **other noncommunicable diseases**, national diabetes programmes were set up in three countries and are under preparation for all European Member States. Continued support is given to research on diabetes and atherosclerosis. A global strategy for management of asthma is being developed. Community-oriented programmes for the control of rheumatic diseases were expanded to five countries, and WHO's recommendations on prevention of rheumatic fever/rheumatic heart disease are already being applied in 24 countries. Health education booklets on this subject were published.

Mental health

Guidelines were issued on primary prevention of mental retardation, epilepsy and suicide and on the use of essential treatments in psychiatry. An assessment of the burden on relatives of caring for a demented person at home was undertaken. Booklets were produced on family care of a relative with Alzheimer disease and with schizophrenia. Psychological problems seen in primary health care were studied with a view to developing treatment guidelines, as were the long-term course and outcome of schizophrenia, obsessive-compulsive and other disorders. Clinical descriptions and diagnostic guidelines for the mental and behavioural disorders section of the International Classification of Diseases (ICD-10) have now been translated into 18 languages and their dissemination and application promoted. Guidelines were produced on life-skills education in schools and on stimulation by carers during early childhood.

An international review of mental health legislation was undertaken. Methods for assessing systems of mental health care were developed. A series of national and regional meetings on neurology and public health was initiated. The network of health authorities on support and rehabilitation of people disabled by chronic mental illness continued to provide guidance in this field. National and regional seminars on diagnostic guidelines and criteria were organized and training workshops held for researchers on the use of WHO interview schedules.

Substance abuse

WHO maintains constant vigilance over the abuse potential of psychoactive substances. As part of a mechanism in effect since 1949, a WHO expert committee reviewed data on selected psychoactive substances and issued advice on the need for regulatory control. Rational prescription of psychotropic pharmaceutical products is being

Support has been given for the implementation of national cancer pain relief and palliative care policies in over 46 countries.

promoted in a number of developing and central and eastern European countries, and a programme on rapid assessment of substance abuse launched in selected African countries. The first phase of a project on drug injection and health risks in 13 countries was completed. Work is proceeding with UNDCP and ILO in five countries on a project dealing with alcohol and drug abuse in the workplace, and with UNHCR on approaches to the prevention of substance abuse among refugees. Research continues on problems of drugs and sports and the social and economic consequences of drug abuse. Support is given to Mem-

---

Box 13. *Effective influenza vaccines*

Every year WHO calls a meeting which makes recommendations as to the composition of the influenza vaccine for use in the forthcoming epidemiological season. These recommendations enable manufacturers to produce the correct type of trivalent influenza vaccine which will be used as of September/October in the same year and thanks to which countless lives — and hospital days and workdays — are saved each year.

The influenza virus is a master at disguising itself by rapidly changing parts of its genetic material. Occasionally a completely new subtype appears, triggering a worldwide pandemic, as in 1918, 1957 and 1968; but even small changes in the virus can cause severe epidemics. Since 1933, when the virus was first grown, only four subtypes of human influenza virus have been identified.

Vaccines which are not close to the strain of virus currently in circulation are of low efficiency. The virus is therefore kept under high surveillance by WHO, through a worldwide network of 118 national influenza centres in 81 countries. These centres isolate the virus from suspected influenza cases, determine what type it is and follow the spread and the gravity of the disease by monitoring, for instance, absenteeism in industry and schools and trends in mortality. International compatibility is ensured because all centres use diagnostic kits which are distributed by WHO free of charge each year.

The national centres also send samples of the isolated strains to one of three WHO collaborating centres in Australia, the United Kingdom and the USA, where they are received within one or two days. Each keeps a collection of reagents to many variants of the virus, allowing a comparison of their antigenic character. Information from the national centres and the collaborating centres is sent to WHO headquarters where it is collated and published in the *Weekly epidemiological record*. In cases of emergency, such as the isolation of a new type of virus, the information is sent to all Member States by fax, telex or telegraph. A weekly influenza update is available on the WHO computer server.

---

ber States in reviewing policies and legislation on treatment and rehabilitation for drug and alcohol dependence, in elaborating techniques for substance abuse prevention, and in providing ad-

equate treatment and care through service development, community involvement and action-oriented research. A European alcohol action plan is operational in 44 countries, and action plans including measures on alcohol use are under way in 17 healthy cities.

Women's health

Joint policy statements are being prepared and disseminated with UNICEF and UNFPA on major public health issues of concern to women, including AIDS prevention, female genital mutilation, traditional birth attendants, and breast-feeding and HIV. A global action plan on safe motherhood is being implemented with the World Bank and Mothercare (USA), and national safe motherhood action plans were formulated in 10 countries. A country needs assessment instrument for safe motherhood was devised, and the mother-baby package of cost-effective interventions to reduce maternal and neonatal mortality introduced (*Box 8*). Database systems for monitoring patterns and trends in maternal health are being disseminated. A report on women's health and human rights was issued, and a European women's health forum established. An in-depth analysis was made of the health situation of women in central and eastern Europe. By end 1994, 87 research projects were being funded, many focusing on the main causes of maternal death and disability. Some of the studies seek to determine the feasibility of integrating sexually transmitted disease control activities into family planning services. In May 1994, taking into account WHO research, the United States Food and Drug Administration extended the duration of continuous use of the intrauterine device TCu380A from nine to ten years. Research on the determinants of induced abortion in developing countries showed that it is not restricted to the unmarried but is also used by married women to limit family size in the absence of effective contraception. A project was launched to promote simple methods for the early detection of cancer of the cervix and breast in developing countries, and in Europe a study is under way on self-examination of the breast. Quality indicators for the care of breast cancer patients and for perinatal/obstetric care were developed and tested.

Health of the elderly

WHO activities are primarily directed to facilitate healthy aging and thus enable the aging population to exercise their full potential as a resource in the community. Various WHO divisions carry out activities concerned with aging and health, including those responsible for health research (osteoporosis and older women's health); noncommunicable diseases (home care); cardiovascular diseases (stroke and hypertension control); nutrition (anthropometric measures); occupational health (aging and working capacity); family health (health of older women); cancer and palliative care (home care for terminally-ill cancer patients, quality of life); epidemiological surveillance and statistical services (healthy life expectancy network); mental health (dementia, particularly Alzheimer disease, and the burden of care within the family); quality of life assessment; prevention of blindness; emergency and humanitarian action (rehabilitation/relocation of elderly refugees and survivors of natural and other disasters); and diabetes. Annual immunization against influenza is important for older persons and WHO ensures that the most effective vaccine is available every year (*Box 13*).

Examples of WHO's work include the launching of a multinational collaborative study on predictors of osteoarthritis, and a study on the socio-economic and health status of the elderly in five countries of South-East Asia, which will serve as a useful tool for promoting national strategies and plans for care of the elderly. In pursuance of the United Nations international plan of action on aging, WHO is setting up an integrated programme on aging and health, which will become fully operational in 1996.

General health issues

Programme activities relevant to all age groups concern in particular tropical disease research and control, cholera, zoonoses, accident prevention, rehabilitation, oral health, blindness and deafness.

Disease prevention and control

The WHO global plan of action for the elimination of **leprosy** has been adopted by the endemic countries. All now have national strategies and plans of action to eliminate the disease as a public health problem by the year 2000. WHO closely monitors progress towards elimination of the disease and supports independent evaluation of national programmes. The establishment of such programmes has been instrumental in helping several endemic countries and areas in the Western Pacific to reach the target of less than 1 case per 10 000 persons, and in greatly reducing the leprosy problem in South-East Asia.

1994 marked the 20th anniversary of the **onchocerciasis** control programme in West Africa (OCP) sponsored by UNDP, FAO and the World Bank with WHO as executing agency. The number of donors making long-term commitments to the programme now stands at 21. Larviciding allied with drug treatment has so far succeeded in eliminating the disease as a major public health problem in 11 endemic countries in Africa. In the Americas a multinational, multiagency and multidonor coalition has been established to support and coordinate national plans to combat the disease in the six endemic countries. Outside the OCP area, plans are under way to support onchocerciasis control in the remaining African countries where the disease is a public health problem.

Remarkable progress has been made since programmes for eradication of **dracunculiasis (guinea-worm disease)** first began in the late 1980s and early 1990s; national and international support for eradication measures is manifest. A reliable village-based surveillance system has been implemented, with a

WHO is setting up an integrated programme on aging and health, which will become fully operational in 1996.

monthly reporting system operational in all countries. In Pakistan, compared with 1988 when 400 cases were recorded, no case was reported in 1994. Cameroon is close to having totally eradicated its only active focus; the number of cases fell from 871 in 1989 to 9 in 1994. Effective control measures in Ghana and Nigeria have seen extraordinary reductions in annual incidence, from 833 048 cases in both countries in 1989 to 93 670 in 1993.

By December 1995 it is expected that dracunculiasis will be eliminated from most of the endemic countries and that there will be a 95% reduction from the 1 million estimated cases in 1989, with the exception of Sudan, for which reliable figures are not available.

A campaign to eliminate **Chagas disease** was launched in the Southern Cone of the Americas (Argentina, Brazil, Bolivia, Chile, Paraguay and Uruguay), and is to be coordinated by an intergovernmental control commission. National plans and programmes have been prepared, and four countries have already enacted legislation that makes blood screening for the disease compulsory. WHO is coordinating a multicountry programme and supporting the development of slow-release insecticidal paints which have been shown to be nearly twice as effective as traditional sprays in controlling the triatomine vectors and about half as expensive. Funds are provided for operational research to improve spraying operations and blood bank screening. Interruption of vector and transfusional transmission of Chagas disease has been achieved in Uruguay (1994) and Chile (1995).

Support is given for training in the epidemiology and control of **schistosomiasis**. A new candidate vaccine has been identified, and other antigens are at an advanced stage of development towards human field trials. Mass treatment with praziquantel is an efficient way of controlling schistosomiasis when targeted at schools with the largest number of infected children, and a simple questionnaire has been designed which could help identify them. This approach is being tested in several African coun-

tries. Simultaneous treatment with praziquantel and a broad-spectrum anthelminthic has been demonstrated to be safe. It has also been shown that simultaneous delivery of the drugs reduces the cost and increases the effectiveness of interventions.

Integrated human and animal **trypanosomiasis** programmes were submitted to the European Union for support. Guidelines are being produced on control methods involving community participation. The effectiveness of seven-day treatments with eflornithine was demonstrated. The drug is expensive, but WHO was able to provide it to four countries on a cost-recovery basis. A low-cost synthesis and production method is being developed.

WHO together with UNICEF provided emergency supplies for serological diagnosis and drug treatment of visceral **leishmaniasis** during a recent epidemic in Sudan. A surveillance system involving a network of 14 institutions in the Mediterranean basin was set up to cope with the emerging problem of HIV/*Leishmania* co-infections. A standardized case report form and guidelines for diagnosis and treatment were prepared.

Guidelines for implementation of the global **malaria** control strategy were produced and adapted to regional needs. Already 25 of the 45 malaria endemic countries of Africa have drawn up plans of action and 10 are implementing them according to the strategy. WHO in collaboration with other agencies and NGOs responded promptly to requests for assistance to combat epidemics in seven countries, including epidemics among 500 000 Rwandan refugees. Guidelines on diagnosis and treatment of malaria in Africa were produced and distributed in French, English and Portuguese.

Progress has been made in many countries towards the required reorientation of their national programmes in line with the global strategy, although the process of reorientation of programmes in the Eastern Mediterranean is being seriously hampered by political instability and wars in a number of countries.

By December 1995 it is expected that dracunculiasis will be eliminated from most of the endemic countries.

Whilst most countries in the Americas have made major steps in integrating the traditional malaria control organization into the general health services at the central level, integration at local level has been attempted in only a few such as Brazil, Colombia, Honduras and Nicaragua. Several countries in the Americas have had to revise their legislation to allow for the integration of services and to promote intersectoral collaboration.

In view of the rapid spread of chloroquine-resistant and multidrug-resistant falciparum malaria, a long-term multicentre collaborative research programme was initiated to study ways of retarding further development of drug resistance. The status of resistance is continuously monitored in all the malarious countries of South-East Asia.

The integration of malaria control with the strategy of primary health care varies in the Western Pacific, in keeping with the way each country has built up its primary health care activities. Integration with the general health services exists in several countries but there are problems at the periphery where workers have difficulties in giving time to the necessary health education and preventive measures.

The synthetic Colombian malaria vaccine, SPf66, has been extensively studied in South America and more recently in Africa and South-East Asia (see *Box 14*). It has given promising results in studies in the United Republic of Tanzania. Multicentre field trials of insecticide-treated bednets are under way in four African countries to assess their effect in reducing mortality in children under age 5. A multicentre field study was initiated to validate a newly developed dip-stick method for detection of falciparum malaria.

Guidelines for the diagnosis, treatment and control of **dengue** and **dengue haemorrhagic fever** were finalized, and national prevention and control strategies are being prepared. With support from WHO, Mahidol University in Bangkok developed a tetravalent live-attenuated dengue vaccine. Clinical trials have shown that it is safe and the immunological response encouraging,

and it is hoped that it will be ready for phase III (efficacy) testing shortly.

The public health implications of lymphatic **filariasis** are being assessed, and pilot control programmes initiated in some countries. Multicentre field trials of ivermectin and new regimes of diethylcarbamazine citrate (DEC) showed the two drugs to be equally effective. Antibiotics, antifungal agents and simple local hygiene were found to reduce elephantiasis.

Box 14. Malaria vaccines

A number of vaccines of potential value in controlling malaria are currently under development. Asexual blood-stage vaccines are designed to reduce severe and complicated manifestations of the disease. They could lower morbidity and mortality in African children under age 5, a particularly high-risk group, and their development is therefore given priority by WHO. A second type of vaccine is designed to arrest the development of the parasite in the mosquito and thus reduce or eliminate transmission of the disease. Research on both types of vaccines is being supported by UNDP/World Bank/WHO.

Asexual blood-stage vaccines are based on antigens derived from the blood stages of *Plasmodium falciparum* present in man. Several are being studied. Together with WHO and USAID, the European Union has established a malaria antigen database for use throughout the world through the Internet. In addition collaborative efforts are under way in the USA to purify sufficient amounts of merozoite surface protein 1, an antigen which has been shown to protect monkeys from infection. Clinical trials using this material could be initiated by late 1995. Trials of two other leading recombinant candidate vaccine antigens, serine rich antigen and an apical membrane antigen, could begin in 1996.

A synthetic "cocktail" vaccine for *P. falciparum*, called SPf66 and developed by Dr M. Patarroyo in Colombia, has been tested extensively in South America and more recently in Africa and South-East Asia. This vaccine, formulated as a peptide-alum combination, was selected for clinical studies on the basis of its ability to protect monkeys from infection. A recent field study among children under age 5 in the United Republic of Tanzania showed that the vaccine was safe, induced antibodies and reduced the risk of developing clinical malaria by about 30%. These findings together with the results from South America confirmed the potential of the vaccine to confer partial protection in areas of high as well as low transmission. Other studies in the Gambia in toddlers aged 6-11 months and in Thailand in children aged 2-15 years are due to be completed by mid-1995.

A meeting to review all the available data on SPf66 will be held in September 1995. It will then be decided whether to undertake further studies to determine its potential for reducing malaria mortality and complications in African children under age 5. If a significant reduction in mortality is observed, registration of the vaccine would proceed.

As far as transmission blocking vaccines are concerned, Pfs25 is a leading candidate and a preparation based on it should go into clinical trials in the USA and Africa during 1995.

Any effective malaria vaccine approved for large-scale application would be used as part of integrated malaria control measures including other protective interventions and disease management.

WHO's global task force on **cholera** control, with the collaboration of the Swiss Disaster Relief Unit and the governments of Australia and Italy, continued to support activities to strengthen countries' capacity to prepare for and respond to epidemics of cholera and dysentery. Multidisciplinary teams were sent to help combat outbreaks of cholera in Somalia and of cholera and dysentery among Rwandan refugees in Zaire. WHO supports a laboratory surveillance system for monitoring drug resistance in the causative organisms that is available to all the cholera-prone countries in Africa, the Eastern Mediterranean and South-East Asia.

Several vaccines are at different stages of development. Grants were provided to Myanmar, Nepal, Sri Lanka and Thailand for strengthening their laboratory capabilities to isolate and characterize *Vibrio cholerae* strains which first appeared in southern India towards the end of 1992. A grant was given to India for large-scale production of O139 antiserum, which was made available to all the cholera-prone countries in Africa, the Eastern Mediterranean and South-East Asia. Because of the potential of the new strain to cause another pandemic, national diarrhoeal disease programme managers, government officials, scientists, and staff from WHO and UNICEF made an in-depth review of the situation.

Global surveillance of emerging and re-emerging **zoonoses** such as rabies, salmonellosis, echinococcosis, liver fluke infection and salmonellosis is being strengthened, and research and technology transfer coordinated. A variety of training courses, consultations and workshops are organized regionally and interregionally.

Oral health

A global data bank is maintained, and support given for situation analyses and the formulation of national plans to promote oral health. WHO participated in the launching of a district-based oral health project in 8 countries. A study on oral health outcomes was completed in 6 countries using a single protocol

linking sociological and clinical data. An international collaborative oral health research initiative is being launched in collaboration with the International Dental Federation, the International Association for Dental Research and the International Federation of Dental Education Associations. An international action network was established on noma and other mutilating diseases and accidents of the face and mouth in African countries. New technologies were introduced for treating dental caries without a drill, water or electricity.

Accidents, violence and suicide

Guides on burn prevention and management are being produced with the International Society for Burn Injuries, and multicentre epidemiological studies on brain injury conducted. A network of demonstration projects on community safety was expanded to 13 countries, and a WHO initiative on spinal cord injury prevention launched. Training materials on injury prevention are being produced, and methodologies for risk assessment continuously monitored and updated.

There has been a significant improvement in meeting the rehabilitation needs of the 35 million persons with disabilities in Africa, using the community-based district health approach pioneered by WHO. Consultant services were provided in 10 countries on programme planning or evaluation, and plans drawn up on strengthening services for refugees and people living in slums. Two intercountry workshops were organized on the management and review of rehabilitation programmes.

Blindness and deafness

Global data on blindness were updated. Quality standards were prepared for small-scale manufacturers of intraocular implants used in cataract surgery. Joint action with NGOs was strengthened through the establishment of a task force on coordination, and extrabudgetary funding mobilized to provide technical support. Advocacy for blind-

Teams were sent to help combat outbreaks of cholera in Somalia and of cholera and dysentery among Rwandan refugees in Zaire.

ness prevention was strengthened in collaboration with the International Council of Ophthalmology and the International Agency for the Prevention of Blindness.

Technical support was provided for workshops on the formulation and management of programmes for prevention and treatment of deafness. Awareness of the problem and the need for action was promoted in collaboration with Hearing International.

Lifestyles and environment

Two of the changes needed to achieve health for all are concerned with a healthy environment and healthy lifestyles and require initiatives by the individual, the family and the community. Activities are carried out in the areas of mental health, healthy public policy, social support systems, healthy living, tobacco, alcohol and psychoactive drug use as well as housing, pollution and food safety. Many of the measures require government involvement at central, regional and local levels and well-integrated, multisectoral planning and management.

WHO promotes *healthy lifestyles* by mobilizing public opinion and the media and strengthening health education and advocacy for health. A school health education resource centre and database were developed, and two regional networks of health promoting schools established. The health promoting schools project established in Europe in 1992 now covers 28 countries. The regions for health network in Europe, founded in 1992, was expanded to include 20 regions.

Global data on *tobacco* are systematically collected, computerized and distributed. Support is given for the development and monitoring of national tobacco control programmes. Within the framework of the European action plan for a tobacco-free Europe, agreement was reached to use tobacco control laws and litigation as public health tools. The Winter Olympic Games in Lillehammer (Norway) were smoke-free as a result of collaboration between the International Olympic Committee and WHO. The theme of the 1994 WHO World No-Tobacco Day, "The media and tobacco: getting the health message across", was widely picked up by the media, thanks to national and local activities around the world.

"Africa 2000", a new investment initiative aimed at providing universal coverage of *water supply and sanitation* services, was launched. A broad programme for hygiene education and promotion of low-cost sanitation is being developed in cooperation with UNICEF and other bilateral and multilateral organizations. Key hygiene behaviours and principles for promoting sanitation were identified. Modules for water supply, sanitation and disposal of solid wastes were developed for UNRWA, and WHO/FAO/UNEP collaborative research initiatives were launched with regional research agencies. A joint project is under way with the United States Environmental Protection Agency to strengthen environmental monitoring and legislation in small communities. Training packages and manuals on the proper operation, maintenance and optimization of systems are being prepared, and one on health in water resources development is being tested.

In the field of *urban health* the global network of healthy cities has been expanded in all regions, and now includes over 650 cities. At the same time close partnership has been established with the OECD ecological cities project. The healthy cities project, launched by WHO, has proved highly effective in mobilizing action on alcohol, HIV/AIDS, diabetes, disability, health-promoting hospitals, nutrition, primary health care, tobacco-free cities, sports, the unemployed, and women and health. Support is given in strengthening national mechanisms for priority-setting, planning and local environmental health research.

The global WHO/UNEP networks for air and water quality monitoring are operational in more than 60 countries, and a comprehensive report on urban

The global network of healthy cities has been expanded in all regions, and now includes over 650 cities.

Box 15. Food safety

Foodborne diseases result from contamination of food with bacterial, viral, parasitic or chemical agents. Although no precise information is available, the problem of food contamination and foodborne diseases can be estimated to be immense on the basis of data on the incidence of diarrhoeal diseases. In addition to acute symptoms, contaminants of food can cause severe and chronic health problems, which are less well known. Some foodborne trematodes are believed to be the underlying factor in liver cancer. Salmonellosis and campilobacteriosis have been found to cause reactive arthritis in some subjects. Enterohaemorrhagic *Escherichia coli* can cause severe disorders of the renal system. Listeriosis and toxoplasmosis are particularly dangerous during pregnancy, as they can be fatal to the fetus, or may result in severe deformity. Heavy metals, like lead, can severely affect the nervous system. Foodborne diseases can lead to severe growth faltering. Infants and children become less resistant to other infections and are caught in a vicious downward spiral of infection and malnutrition leading in many cases to death. Foodborne diseases incur tremendous economic costs in terms both of reduced productivity and of medical care. During the 1991 cholera epidemic Peru had to sustain medical care costs for the thousands of people affected. In addition its food exports decreased substantially and its tourism industry was affected.

Food can become contaminated at any stage in the food chain, from production to processing and handling prior to consumption. Therefore the causes of foodborne diseases tend to be multiple and interdependent. In developing countries lack of basic sanitation and use of untreated night-soil as fertilizer or untreated wastewater for irrigation allow pathogens to be introduced into the food chain through the water. In developed countries improved standards of living have led to a rise in consumption of food of animal origin. The resulting mass production of animals has increased the risk that many will be subclinically infected with foodborne pathogens such as *Salmonella* and *Campylobacter*. Research continues under WHO auspices on the uses of irradiation and modern biotechnology to improve the food supply.

Traditions and beliefs also contribute to the occurrence of foodborne diseases in both developed and developing countries. For example in some cultures raw meat products, raw fish or raw milk are traditional foods, despite the health risks. Finally some diseases are imported from endemic areas because of the growing number of international travellers, for whom WHO has published a popular guide.

Because of its role in the spread of contaminants, the Codex Alimentarius system was set up to facilitate world trade in food, promote fair practices and protect consumers by establishing internationally accepted standards. Standards are set in such areas as maximum allowed amounts of pesticide residues and contaminants in raw materials, labelling of food and maximum content of approved food additives, in addition to codes of hygienic and technological practice. Application of the standards not only protects the health of consumers, but avoids the temptation to use health-related national standards as an excuse for unfair trade practices. The standards are set by the Codex Alimentarius Commission which is jointly sponsored by FAO and WHO. It works by harmonizing national standards in consultation with governments, trade and industry representatives, consumers' associations and others. Some 200 standards and 140 codes and guidelines have been published in 25 volumes in 3 languages. Until recently these instruments were sent to governments as recommendations for action. With the signature of the Final Act of the Uruguay Round of multilateral trade negotiations launched by GATT, those related to food safety became internationally recognized reference values.

air quality in megacities was published. Surface- and ground-water quality are monitored in over 350 cities worldwide, and several methodology guidelines were issued on sampling and analysis of air and water. The distribution of revised WHO guidelines for drinking-water quality was followed by a series of national and regional seminars to stimulate the enactment and application of standards at national level. Guidelines for the safe handling and disposal of hospital and other infectious wastes are being prepared.

The major thrust for WHO activities in the sphere of *food safety* is to support the adoption of modern food safety strategies that no longer rely exclusively on end-product testing but rather focus on monitoring "critical control points" in food production and processing and on promoting awareness of problems and stimulating information development and transfer. WHO takes a multidisciplinary and multisectoral approach to the prevention of foodborne diseases (*Box 15*). Two new collaborating centres for food safety were designated, and several projects implemented. Risk assessment of chemicals in food is being strengthened, and food contamination by heavy metals, industrial chemicals and pesticides monitored through a joint UNEP/FAO/WHO programme. Together with FAO, WHO has established acceptable daily intakes for well over 700 food additives, contaminants and veterinary drug residues in food. WHO cosponsors regional and subregional courses and workshops on food safety. WHO and FAO support the Codex Alimentarius Commission, an intergovernmental body with a current membership of 146 countries, which encourages the development of scientifically-based and internationally-agreed food standards. The recently concluded Uruguay Round of multilateral trade negotiations recognizes Codex standards, guidelines and recommendations as international reference values to ensure that unnecessary or overly restrictive requirements are not used as non-tariff barriers to international trade.

Health infrastructure

Coverage, accessibility and quality of care are three basic requirements in health development. Coverage depends on the availability of suitably located facilities where quality care is given to the whole population by well-trained health workers using appropriate technologies. Many problems have been encountered in building up health infrastructures, ranging from lack of clear national policies and leadership, to inadequate resources and bad management.

Health services worldwide are being reformed to meet the challenges forced on countries by dramatic economic and social changes. The reforms are to the extent possible based on the primary health care approach, are in line with global, regional and national health-for-all strategies and are designed to ensure equity in health care, allied with greater efficiency and effectiveness. Specific activities are concerned with the organization of health systems based on primary health care; the development of human resources for health; clinical, laboratory and radiological technology; the provision of essential drugs; drug and vaccine quality, safety and efficacy; and traditional medicine.

As part of its support to governments in the organization of **health systems based on primary health care**, WHO provides them with updated information on ways to manage change. It advises on particular aspects of reform such as the appropriate mix of public and private services, decentralization, and effective links between central authorities, district health systems and local communities. It helps health policymakers to identify priority areas. In the Western Pacific, for example, a forum was organized to enable countries to share experiences in health development; and support was given to several South-East Asian countries in formulating new health policies and strategies as part of a reorganization of their health systems. In Europe urgent attention was paid to the revitalization and modern-ization of sometimes inefficient, unbalanced and inert medical care systems. Emphasis was placed on attracting more financial resources, decentralizing and dismantling monolithic top-down structures, remotivating health care workers, and making systems more rational, efficient and responsive to consumers. A manual on a "basic minimum needs" kit was produced and will be issued in the near future. A national quality assurance system was established in Saudi Arabia and is being introduced in other Eastern Mediterranean countries. Saudi Arabia, with WHO support, published four reference manuals on quality of health care, dealing with primary health care, nursing, health inspection and pharmacy. These documents have been widely distributed and adopted by other Member States. WHO collaborates with a number of countries in the Eastern Mediterranean in improving national health information systems and establishing the managerial process for health development.

Health care financing systems are being restructured in several countries in the Americas, and application of the "basic minimum needs" approach is being accelerated. There are moves to expand the role of the private sector in the provision of health care in South-East Asia. Generally people are becoming increasingly interested in the services they receive and pay for, either as consumers or as taxpayers. Greater attention is being given to the financing of health systems in the Western Pacific. Experiments are under way with insurance schemes, public or private partnership, incentive payments, cost sharing and cost recovery.

In the Western Pacific the primary health care approach is being adapted to address new challenges. Priority is given to emerging health needs in connection with urbanization, environmental change and chronic diseases associated with lifestyle. Countries in South-East Asia are strengthening their district health systems based on primary health care with emphasis on reaching underserved and unserved populations.

> *Health services worldwide are being reformed to meet the challenges forced on countries by dramatic economic and social changes.*

Community involvement in health now seems to be widely accepted in most countries.

All African countries have adopted and are implementing the African health development framework, whereby community-oriented, locally managed activities are carried out with appropriate support from district, intermediate and central levels of the health system and other sectors. There is now a consensus that a well-defined district health-for-all package, with specified minimum activities, is a good tool for extending services beyond simple curative care to include health promotion and prevention.

Through research and direct support of countries, WHO actively promotes **community involvement in health** aimed at enabling people to take responsibility for decisions concerning their health and to make their health services more effective. Community involvement in health now seems to be widely accepted in most countries. It finds its expression in such ways as ensuring equitable and rational distribution of resources for health; mobilizing funds from local, national and international sources; and making good use of the knowledge and experience available within the community. The topic of community action for health was extensively discussed by the World Health Assembly in 1994.

As part of efforts for the development of **human resources for health**, WHO launched an initiative to determine optimum approaches to the training of health personnel under changing socioeconomic conditions. In the Americas emphasis is given to the management of education programmes for the medical and related professions. WHO is devising tools for policy analysis and planning in the Eastern Mediterranean and South-East Asia. It collaborates with countries in reviewing health personnel policies and plans within the perspective of existing economic constraints. In the Western Pacific several reviews of public health training and medical education were carried out; they highlighted the need to reorient health personnel planning and training to the requirements of health development over the next five

years. WHO continued its efforts to enhance national capabilities to design and implement appropriate programmes for medical, nursing and other health personnel, and gave intensified support to national educational institutions. WHO fellowships are being monitored and evaluated to ensure that they are relevant to national health-for-all strategies.

National action plans on nursing and midwifery are being prepared together with a plan for regional and interregional action in support of WHO's goals through collaborating centres. Strategies are being developed to upgrade the quality of nursing practice through networks of chief nursing officers. A meeting of chief nursing/midwifery officers, educators and managers from eastern and southern Africa was held to discuss ways to give nurses and midwives a greater role in improving health care at district level. WHO collaborates with the International Confederation of Nurses, the International Confederation of Midwives and other NGOs in this field. Microcomputer-based models for projecting staff availability and requirements are being field-tested, using workload indicators to determine staffing need. A guide on functional job analysis is being prepared.

WHO plays a central role in promoting **health technology** assessment in developing countries, particularly in relation to primary health care, disease prevention and control, nutrition and environmental health. Materials produced on this subject included a handbook of principles for the management of radiological services; guidelines for planning and organization of small imaging departments; new technical specifications for the WHO radiographic unit as part of the WHO imaging system; a set of standard radiographs for reference use in small hospitals and radiology practices; and a manual on radiation protection in hospitals and general practice. Basic safety standards on radiation protection and radiation sources are being established with FAO, IAEA, ILO and OECD. A number of studies were carried out on development of a standard cold chain for blood; the incidence of HIV following blood transfusion; and inactivation of viruses in blood products. Portable laboratory instruments and photovoltaic equipment are being tested, and field trials of an oxygen concentrator machine that meets WHO specifications conducted jointly with the World Federation of Societies of Anaesthesiologists. A new training centre on repair and maintenance of medical equipment is being set up in the Syrian Arab Republic in collaboration with UNDP.

In the field of *pharmaceuticals* the Organization collaborates with national drug regulatory authorities in harmonizing approaches to drug registration and surveillance, establishing international standards for quality assurance, and exchanging information on national regulatory decisions. The rational use of drugs can be ensured only within a well-defined framework of regulation. Through its model lists and related prescribing information, WHO helps countries to foster cost-effective drug use and procurement. Activities concerned with the promotion of national drug policy are described in the following section, under *Health policy*.

The WHO model list of *essential drugs*, which helps countries to match priority drugs to priority health needs, is revised and updated biennially. Collation of an international database on suspected adverse drug reactions continues. The content and scope of WHO's model prescribing information are being expanded, its ethical criteria for medicinal drug promotion reviewed, and its recommended good practices in the manufacture and quality control of drugs updated. Pharmacopoeial standards and other requirements for pharmaceutical and biological products continue to be established, and international nonproprietary names for pharmaceutical substances selected.

A model software package was produced to support drug registration using a desk-top computer. Basic tests are being devised to verify the identity of pharmaceutical substances outside a laboratory setting. Good manufacturing practices have been extensively revised, and proposals formulated for the registration of generic products. Guidelines for implementation of the WHO Certification Scheme on the Quality of Pharmaceutical Products moving in International Commerce are being field-tested.

WHO assists in incorporating *traditional medicine* into national health systems in countries where it is widely practised, and promotes operational research, clinical investigations and exchange of information on the subject. A comparative review is being made of legislation on traditional and alternative medicine, and guidelines prepared on safe techniques and basic training in acupuncture. A study is under way on the indications and contraindications of acupuncture.

Health policy

The most important way in which WHO influences national health development is by helping to shape health policy. The Organization works closely with Member countries in analysing and designing policies concerned with health, helps strengthen national managerial capabilities, supports countries in implementing and evaluating their national health-for-all strategies, and advises on the application of health information systems. Technical support is given in formulating policy relating to health legislation, drugs and environmental health, including assessment of the risk of potentially toxic chemicals.

A major step was taken in the area of *women, health and development*. In 1993 the Global Commission on Women's Health was established as an advisory body to WHO. It drew up an agenda for action on women's health covering nutrition, reproductive health, the health consequences of violence, aging, lifestyle-related conditions and the work environment. It has raised awareness among policy-makers of women's health issues and encourages their inclusion in all development plans as a priority. A report on women's health

The most important way in which WHO influences national health development is by helping to shape health policy.

and human rights, drafted for the 1993 World Conference on Human Rights in Vienna, was published. Under the auspices of the commission, a scheme to provide credit and banking facilities to the most vulnerable and disadvantaged is being implemented in Africa. At the 1994 International Conference on Population and Development in Cairo, WHO played a key role in helping to reach consensus and transcend political and religious differences. This was made possible by WHO's inclusive approach to health, which is unique both within the United Nations system and globally. Where other agencies may be concerned with single issues, products or interventions in the health field, proposals by WHO receive high marks for both medical and ethical credibility because of its nonpartisan and priority concern for the overall health and well-being of all individuals in all societies.

WHO's activities relating to *environment, health and development* stem in particular from the agreement reached at the 1992 United Nations Conference on Environment and Development (UNCED) that countries should prepare and implement national plans for sustainable development. A major interregional WHO/UNDP initiative seeks to promote the incorporation of health and environment concerns in the plans. So far financial and technical support has been provided to six countries for that purpose. WHO has been designated task manager for the "health chapter" of UNCED. WHO in collaboration with several United Nations bodies prepared a progress report on health, environment and sustainable development, stressing the importance of reform with respect to community development, environmental health, national decision-making and national accounting. Health indicators in relation to sustainable development are being established.

In pursuance of the new global strategy on health and environment, several WHO regional offices drew up corresponding regional strategies and action plans. A second European Conference on Environment and Health in Helsinki

in 1994 endorsed an environmental health action plan for Europe and outlined in the Helsinki Declaration a mechanism for long-term cooperation between the major players in this field. In the Western Pacific the impact of development on health was evaluated using environmental assessment guidelines. Support was given for the formulation of environmental health action plans in areas with high development potential, and national capabilities for preparing such plans were strengthened.

Materials produced by WHO included guidelines on the operation of poisons control facilities, 15 health and safety guides, and over 200 international chemical safety cards providing basic information on the diagnosis and treatment of poisonings. A global database on chemical substances, pharmaceuticals, poisonous plants and animals was issued; and intercountry training workshops on prevention and treatment of poisonings and on chemical safety were organized. Together with WMO and UNEP, WHO is studying the health impact of ozone layer depletion and analysing the potential health impact of global climate change.

As part of efforts for *strengthening of national managerial capabilities* WHO is providing support to enable 26 countries in greatest need to formulate and implement health reform policies, draw up plans for correcting inequities, improve the financing and management of health systems, mobilize resources and make more effective use of external funds.

WHO coordinates aid for strategic health reform and facilitates the process in individual countries. For instance support was provided to Mozambique, Nepal, Sierra Leone and Viet Nam in dealing with health economics and financing; to Zambia in setting up health reform teams and designing methodology; and to Bolivia, Guatemala and Guinea-Bissau in strengthening district health systems.

WHO's EUROHEALTH programme, set up in 1991, is a blueprint for use by countries in mobilizing the internal and external resources needed to redesign their health systems. An

At the 1994 International Conference on Population and Development in Cairo, WHO played a key role in helping to reach consensus and transcend political and religious differences.

external evaluation of the programme showed that it has been successful in supporting countries in need. Helping countries to prepare a framework for international collaboration along the lines of health for all is now considered more important than ever.

By the end of 1994 WHO was present in all the new independent states with 21 WHO liaison offices in operation. Support was provided for fund-raising, health care reform, procurement of pharmaceuticals and vaccines, and implementation of programmes in such areas as immunization and maternal and child health including family planning and breast-feeding. Medium-term collaboration programmes were prepared for new independent states and for Israel, Malta and Turkey. An expert network on health care financing strategies placed specialized knowledge at the disposal of new independent states and influenced the direction of their reforms and health legislation. A WHO advisory group on health care reforms in Europe was set up.

WHO works with bilateral agencies, other United Nations bodies and NGOs in developing national **drug policy** frameworks and collaborates with 55 countries on such questions as drug selection, legislation, manufacture and quality assurance. National drug policies were formulated in Egypt and Yemen and existing policies reviewed in Sudan and Tunisia. WHO promotes North-South transfer of drug production technology as well as quality assurance and good manufacturing practices, particularly in Africa and South-East Asia. A list of life-saving drugs was prepared and is proving valuable in new independent states which have suffered acute shortages.

Policy-related operational research projects are being implemented on the financing, management and rational use of drugs and vaccines, and studies continue on the impact of the private sector on drug supply, and on measures to stimulate the availability of generic essential drugs. Findings were disseminated through universities, networks

and publications. Guidelines, tools and training materials were distributed on such topics as policy and management, supply and logistics, quality assurance and rational drug use.

WHO facilitates access to a number of databases through WHO Gopher, World Wide Web and Telnet. These contain **information** on WHO and its programmes, press releases and specific technical data on such subjects as communicable diseases and HIV/AIDS. Through the Internet facility WHO has established several bulletin boards on health technology, tools for health research and nursing in the 21st century among others. An international electronic bulletin board capability for discussing health futures was set up. A WHO information centre for health was opened in Kyrgyzstan to serve the central Asian republics.

In collaboration with Member States WHO completed the monitoring of progress towards health for all by the year 2000 and prepared a third report on the findings for submission to the WHO governing bodies in 1995. Country health profiles as well as computerized regional and global health-for-all databases were updated. Support was given to over 30 countries in preparing national language versions of the tenth revision of the International Classification of Diseases (ICD-10) and in implementing the revised classification, particularly by providing guidelines and organizing training courses.

WHO has launched a new health futures research initiative for exploring probable, possible and preferable futures in relation to such issues as the health trends expected in the next millennium and the probable impact on health of technologies that are likely to emerge during the next decade. Some of the methods were considered at a 1993 WHO consultation on health futures methodology, and results are now being assessed in countries for their relevance and feasibility. Findings are shared through a network of over 300 experts on health monitoring, evaluation and futures studies.

A list of life-saving drugs has been prepared and is proving valuable in new independent states which have suffered acute shortages.

Periodically WHO assesses the global health situation and trends for some priority diseases and conditions and disseminates the findings through publications, for instance dealing with the world health situation and projections. Following a decision by the WHO Executive Board in 1994 concerning the recommendations of its working group on the WHO response to global change, steps were taken to make annual assessments of global health status and trends and to issue the findings as from 1995. The present publication, *The World Health Report 1995 – bridging the gaps*, was prepared in response to that decision.

Coordination

WHO's coordination activities involve support to sessions of the WHO governing bodies, partnership with other United Nations organizations, international development agencies and NGOs, mobilization of external resources, emergency relief operations, food aid and public relations. Highlights of WHO's collaboration with international and regional development agencies are given below.

The continuing crisis of development in Africa was recognized as one of the greatest challenges facing the **United Nations system** and the entire international community. WHO's major input was channelled through humanitarian programmes coordinated by the United Nations Department of Humanitarian Affairs and funded from consolidated appeals as well as the Central Emergency Revolving Fund (CERF). Appeals for financing health work were usually less well supported than other components, but WHO continued to stress the strong interrelationship between all aspects of humanitarian activities and the importance of linking emergency relief to reconstruction and development.

The growing awareness among Member States of the need to improve health care delivery systems, and a notable interest on the part of the **World**

Bank to promote improvements in the social sector, provided a timely opportunity to forge closer links between WHO, the Bank and governments.

Joint collaboration with **UNICEF** focused on the 21 goals related to the health of women and children in the plan of action adopted at the 1990 World Summit for Children. The UNICEF/WHO Joint Committee on Health Policy reviewed progress with respect to the mid-decade summit goals (1995).

WHO cooperates with **FAO** in helping countries to consolidate their national plans of action for nutrition, as recommended in the 1992 World Declaration and Plan of Action for Nutrition. Joint meetings were organized in three regions and plans made to hold similar meetings in two further regions in early 1995.

The greater emphasis given to the social sector by the five **United Nations regional commissions** provided an opportunity for WHO to reinforce its relations with these organizations and to strengthen coordination of its work with other United Nations bodies. WHO collaborated with the Economic and Social Commission for Asia and the Pacific on such subjects as environment and sustainable development, HIV/AIDS, preventable diseases, disability and population.

Cooperation with the Commission of the **European Union** on emergency and humanitarian assistance to the countries of former Yugoslavia was intensified, with about one-third of the resources available for WHO activities coming from the commission. The Council of Ministers held two sessions on the European Union's "health in development" policies.

Together with the **Organization of African Unity** and other institutions, WHO pursued the priority objective of supporting African recovery and development. It assisted OAU in formulating a draft health protocol for the treaty establishing the African Economic Community (the Abuja treaty of 1991), which will provide a framework for health and development in Africa as a

> The continuing crisis of development in Africa is one of the greatest challenges facing the United Nations system and the entire international community.

whole. Other subjects of collaboration with OAU included a declaration on AIDS and the child in Africa; control of malaria; and a common position on disaster reduction in Africa.

In recent years WHO has significantly strengthened its collaboration with five major *regional development banks*: the African Development Bank, the Asian Development Bank, the European Bank for Reconstruction and Development, the Inter-American Development Bank and the Islamic Development Bank. The banks are giving higher priority to the social sector including health and environmental protection. WHO seeks to provide leadership in health and ensure its inclusion on the agenda of these institutions.

WHO collaborates on an ad hoc basis with a broad range of *nongovernmental organizations*. Formal relations may be established in cases where long-standing and mutually beneficial activities have grown up. In 1994 the number of international NGOs in official relations with WHO reached 184 with the admission of the International Commission on Non-ionizing Radiation Protection, the International Consultation on Urological Diseases, the International Council for Control of Iodine Deficiency Disorders, the International Occupational Hygiene Association, the International Society for Preventive Oncology and the International Society of Surgery. With such partners WHO on the one hand reaches out to put iodized salt on a family table, alert governments and occupational groups to the need for adequate health protection and promotion and ensures that the surgeon's skill is kept properly honed, and on the other serves as a global clearinghouse for exchange of vast amounts of experience and data.

The main objective of WHO's *emergency relief programme* is to strengthen the national capacity of Member States to lessen the adverse health consequences of emergencies and disasters. Activities include the provision of emergency drugs and supplies, the fielding of technical emergency assessment missions and technical support. Emergency

preparedness focuses on coordination, policy-making, awareness-building, technical advice, training, publication of standards and guidelines, and research.

In 1994 WHO provided technical expertise and emergency medical supplies to cope with major natural or man-made disasters in Afghanistan, Angola, Burundi, Iraq, Somalia and Sudan, in former Yugoslavia and in some new independent states. Following outbreaks of cholera, meningitis and malaria in Africa, Europe and Latin America, WHO helped to mobilize international assistance and support for prevention and control.

From the very onset of the crisis in Rwanda, WHO assisted in assessing the situation and the emergency needs arising from it, in close association with the United Nations Department of Humanitarian Affairs. The cooperation grew steadily from April 1994 onwards and WHO is now responsible for providing the required coordination in the health sector, among other things in order to link the initial emergency response to rehabilitation and reconstruction of the health infrastructure throughout the country.

WHO took part in 10 joint missions with WFP concerned with the use of *food aid* in support of human resources development. The Organization's recommendations on prevention of disease and monitoring of disease trends were applied in food-for-work projects.

Publishing, language and library services

Countries throughout the world call on WHO for up-to-date, reliable and authoritative health information. For all of them, the overriding concern is how to obtain the right information at the right time with limited resources. Electronic networks and other modern information technology help to provide new ways of doing this. WHO publishes and distributes books and guidelines on priority health issues, translates essential technical and administrative texts,

The main objective of WHO's emergency relief programme is to strengthen the national capacity of Member States to lessen the adverse health consequences of emergencies and disasters.

and increases worldwide access to health information through libraries and health literature networks. For many health workers in developing countries, WHO materials are often the only source of reliable information on crucial aspects of disease control. For most, it is their only contact with an Organization which is there to serve them. Feedback, especially from developing countries, shows that much of the material, especially from *World health*[f] and *World health forum*, is widely used and reproduced. The combined readership for these two journals and the *Bulletin of the World Health Organization* is estimated at 700 000. The network of sales agents and clients on account now covers over 100 countries, and annual revenue from sales of WHO publications has reached nearly $4 million. This revenue is used to finance the further circulation of WHO books and periodicals to the extent that 80% are distributed free of charge.

General administration

Largely because of the economic climate that has prevailed over the last decade, and a zero or negative growth budget in real terms, a particular concern has been to achieve cost savings and cost avoidance. Bearing in mind the need to limit adverse effects on the Organization's programmes, operations are being streamlined and improved, particularly in the areas of new technology (e.g. introduction of electronic mail facilities, computerization of records management, preparation of inventories of office equipment); contracting out (e.g. grounds maintenance, night security, cleaning); downsizing (e.g. reduction in the frequency of mail distribution); and redistribution of resources (e.g. a shift from administrative to field staff to provide humanitarian assistance). Efforts will continue to identify all possible cost-saving measures while ensuring an acceptable level and quality of service.

Following a reduction in staff at WHO headquarters since 1992, a rationalization of procedures in the Organization's **supply services** has been undertaken. The greater part of WHO's air freight operations have been contracted out. Although the volume of procurement and the number of shipments have increased, because of growing WHO involvement in emergency relief operations, it has been possible to cope with the additional work with a reduced staff thanks to structural changes and improved logistics. Timely arrival of consignments at places which are difficult to access or subject to sanction regulations has been ensured. The standardization of supplies, the development of medical kits and bulk purchasing agreements with suppliers have all led to savings of several million US dollars each year. WHO's performance in providing good quality emergency supplies at competitive cost has encouraged more donors to entrust the Organization with funds. Supply services for relief operations increased during the last two years from less than 10% to almost 20% of the total.

Since 1992 shortfalls in payment of contributions have affected the Organization's situation as regards **finance**. Programme delivery has been ensured by reallocating resources to priority activities and stressing value for money. Improvements in productivity through the use of microcomputers were particularly striking in the Western Pacific.

Emphasis in recruitment of **personnel** has been given to increasing the proportion of women in posts in the professional and higher-graded categories and enhancing the international character of the staff by recruiting from underrepresented countries through active prospection. The number of adequately represented countries increased from 99 in January 1992 to 109 in September 1994. The number of women in the professional and higher-graded categories increased from 382 in September 1992 to 405 in September 1994.

For many health workers in developing countries WHO materials are often the only source of reliable information on crucial aspects of disease control.

[f] The themes of issues in 1994 were oral health; mental health; population; home care; medicine of tomorrow; poverty and health.

Regional highlights[g]

Africa

With the return of South Africa and the affiliation of a new state, Eritrea, the African region now comprises 46 countries. Africa has 29 of the world's 47 least developed countries. The remaining 17 Member States are all developing countries.

Access to health care is generally poor. The region lacks human resources for health, and there has been a constant brain drain which is being exacerbated by the severe economic recession in most Member States. Health infrastructures remain underfunded and poorly managed; coverage, while showing a steady increase, remains inadequate. Referral facilities are poorly staffed and ill-equipped, and neonatal care is often lacking. All the countries of the region have adopted the essential drugs strategy and the majority have their own essential drugs list. However, because of weak purchasing power, there is a constant shortage of standard drugs in the health services.

Per capita expenditure on health is on the whole very low in African countries, ranging from $3.5 to a maximum of $290. The population growth rate of sub-Saharan Africa between 1950 and 1990 was between 2.2% and 3.3%, resulting in an increase from 170 million to 500 million in that period. Women have an average of 6 children, 45% of the population are under age 15, and elderly people of 60 years and above constitute about 5% of the total.

Maternal mortality rates are unacceptably high, ranging from 62 to 1 000 per 100 000 live births. Most women go through childbirth without the benefit of trained assistance.

Although more progress in water supply and sanitation occurred in Africa during the international water supply and sanitation decade than in any other comparable period, to date 52% of the population still lack safe water and 68% are without proper sanitation. There is evidence that 50 million pre-school children suffer from protein-energy malnutrition. Of the 46 capital cities in the region 19 have recently experienced civic unrest, seriously disrupting health services. Peace and security are needed if progress is to be made.

Between 1980 and 1993 the urban population increased at the rate of 5% annually, and the number of city dwellers rose from 83 to 162 million. The obvious result is that municipal authorities cannot adequately meet basic needs in housing, education, health, water supply and waste disposal.

In recent years there have been growing numbers of emergencies associated with natural and man-made disasters, ethnic conflicts and a deteriorating socioeconomic environment. In 1993 close to 16 million Africans were refugees or displaced with attendant health problems including disease outbreaks and malnutrition; 1 million of those suffered severe malnutrition.

Two major initiatives have been launched in the region – the "district health-for-all" package and "Africa 2000", designed to sensitize the international community to the need for adequate water supplies and sanitation.

The polio-free zone in eastern and southern Africa is expanding, and considerable progress has been made towards the elimination of leprosy and dracunculiasis. For many countries, however, falling immunization coverage in the past three years has resulted in increases in the incidence of several diseases. Epidemics of yellow fever, meningitis, cholera and bacillary dysentery have not abated.

Policies, strategies and financial initiatives for primary health care have been accepted in principle by Member States, but they are often difficult to implement. Experience has shown that the key to success lies essentially in good district health management and well-defined priorities.

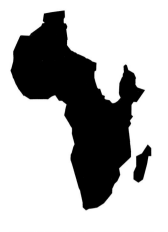

Algeria	Madagascar
Angola	Malawi
Benin	Mali
Botswana	Mauritania
Burkina Faso	Mauritius
Burundi	Mozambique
Cameroon	Namibia
Cape Verde	Niger
Central African Republic	Nigeria
Chad	Rwanda
Comoros	Sao Tome and Principe
Congo	Senegal
Côte d'Ivoire	Seychelles
Equatorial Guinea	Sierra Leone
Eritrea	South Africa
Ethiopia	Swaziland
Gabon	Togo
Gambia	Uganda
Ghana	United Republic of
Guinea	Tanzania
Guinea-Bissau	Zaire
Kenya	Zambia
Lesotho	Zimbabwe
Liberia	

[g] The six WHO regions vary widely in size, socioeconomic development, epidemiological characteristics, culture and history. However, within each of the regions, similar patterns of health development and largely the same health concerns are observed. Highlights are presented in the following pages.

Americas

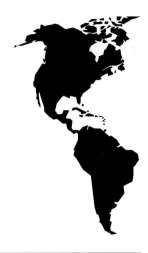

Antigua and Barbuda
Argentina
Bahamas
Barbados
Belize
Bolivia
Brazil
Canada
Chile
Colombia
Costa Rica
Cuba
Dominica
Dominican Republic
Ecuador
El Salvador
Grenada
Guatemala
Guyana
Haiti

Honduras
Jamaica
Mexico
Nicaragua
Panama
Paraguay
Peru
Saint Kitts and Nevis
Saint Lucia
Saint Vincent and the
    Grenadines
Suriname
Trinidad and Tobago
United States of America
Uruguay
Venezuela

Associate Member:
Puerto Rico

The region of the Americas is characterized by great inequalities. The income of the richest 20% of the population is 28 times greater than that of the poorest 20%. In Latin America and the Caribbean 46% of the population live in poverty and half of those, or 100 million people, have no access to either private or public basic health care. Yet almost everywhere, all age groups and both sexes have experienced steadily declining death rates over the last 40 years.

Within countries, however, considerable differentials exist. In line with social and economic inequalities, health systems have tended to concentrate on district and specialist hospitals, providing care to certain social groups and neglecting vast segments of the population, especially the poor.

Urban populations are growing rapidly, creating serious social, health and environmental problems. Environmental and health care deficiencies were harshly illustrated by the cholera epidemic in 1991. Urban and domestic violence is another pressing public health concern in the major cities of the region.

The WHO regional strategy sets out five priority areas for action in 1995-1998. The first is concerned with health in development, with particular attention to policy definition and sectoral reform. The second is strengthening of health systems and services, with emphasis on decentralization and local health systems. Health promotion is the third priority area, focusing on healthy public policies, living conditions, lifestyles, food and nutrition, and the mounting problem of violence. The fourth priority area is environmental health, especially the provision of adequate drinking-water and sanitation. The fifth is control and prevention of diseases, including HIV/AIDS. The region has already been declared free of poliomyelitis, and the elimination of measles, tetanus and foot-and-mouth disease is within reach.

Public health action is targeted towards specific groups such as the elderly and the marginalized poor. Over 400 centres disseminate scientific and technical information as part of a network coordinated by the Regional Library of Medicine in São Paulo (Brazil). Over 12% of the total resources available are allocated to research and especially the improvement of research capacity and training.

The regional programme on bioethics was formally established in 1994, covering the three main areas of public health and health policy; health care particularly in the clinical field; and research and training of researchers. The scope of cooperation activities has been clearly defined. Countries remain the sole point of reference and the basis for the Organization's action. Human, financial, scientific, institutional, moral and political resources are mobilized in several ways with cooperation between countries. Strategic alliances have been set up with multinational financing bodies (which spend over $4 billion per year in support of health activities in the Americas), with the United Nations and inter-American institutions, with bilateral donors and NGOs.

Eastern Mediterranean

Member States of the region share many common features in terms of ethnic composition, language, religion, political tradition, social values and customs. Hence many aspects of social behaviour and mores affecting the health of individuals and communities follow similar patterns. The most commonly spoken language is Arabic, and the most widespread religion is Islam.

At the same time a wide variety of political institutions exist and countries vary considerably in their socioeconomic development. At one end of the spectrum are the politically stable and rich countries with steady, well-coordinated socioeconomic development; in the middle of the spectrum are stable but less rich countries that have been able to sustain reasonable socioeconomic advancement; and at the other end there are poorly-endowed and less stable countries. In these the unsettled political situation, ideological differences, and chronic levels of armed conflict and civil strife severely hamper national development. Similarly, rising military expenditure in a number of countries against a background of economic recession does not make for smooth and unfettered progress.

The impact of inflation and unemployment as well as the continuing decrease in per capita GNP (from $1 375 in 1983 to $1 162 in 1992) has seriously affected the living standards and health status of most people, particularly in the less developed Member States. The total population, about 194 million in 1970, had soared to 298 million by 1984-1985, with an average annual net rate of increase of about 3%.

An epidemiological transition is taking place in the region, with life expectancy at birth gaining 7 years during the last decade, largely due to decreases in infant and childhood mortality.

Coverage with local health services has reached fairly high levels, the regional average being 82%. But the picture varies greatly. Only about half of pregnant women are attended by trained personnel during pregnancy and childbirth, and there has been a slight downward trend during the last few years. Great efforts will be made to reverse it.

In 1993 most countries maintained high levels of immunization of children against vaccine-preventable diseases, and of pregnant women against tetanus. There is clear evidence of significant decreases in these diseases, particularly poliomyelitis. There are already two polio-free zones in the region which have had no or few cases for some years. The rest of the region, apart from war-stricken areas, is following suit.

Countries are universally committed to the cause of health, as witnessed by the immunization carried out in Afghanistan in 1994. The warring factions allowed immunization teams and centres to work in peace and security, leading to hope of a more durable and all-encompassing peace. On another positive note, the Palestine Health Authority started its work in the self-ruled territories. Member States have been called on to provide material and personnel support, in addition to the 1% of the regional budget approved for Palestine.

Several technical guidelines and manuals covering important areas of laboratory and blood transfusion medicine have been produced and a number translated into several languages. Efforts continue towards regional self-sufficiency in quality assurance.

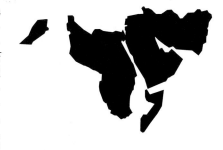

Afghanistan	Morocco
Bahrain	Oman
Cyprus	Pakistan
Djibouti	Qatar
Egypt	Saudi Arabia
Iran (Islamic Republic of)	Somalia
Iraq	Sudan
Jordan	Syrian Arab Republic
Kuwait	Tunisia
Lebanon	United Arab Emirates
Libyan Arab Jamahiriya	Yemen

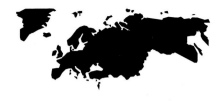

Albania	Malta
Armenia	Monaco
Austria	Netherlands
Azerbaijan	Norway
Belarus	Poland
Belgium	Portugal
Bosnia and Herzegovina	Republic of Moldova
Bulgaria	Romania
Croatia	Russian Federation
Czech Republic	San Marino
Denmark	Slovakia
Estonia	Slovenia
Finland	Spain
France	Sweden
Georgia	Switzerland
Germany	Tajikistan
Greece	The Former Yugoslav
Hungary	Republic of Macedonia
Iceland	Turkey
Ireland	Turkmenistan
Israel	Ukraine
Italy	United Kingdom of
Kazakhstan	Great Britain and
Kyrgyzstan	Northern Ireland
Latvia	Uzbekistan
Lithuania	Yugoslavia
Luxembourg	

Europe

The last few years have witnessed an unprecedented geopolitical transformation in the European region. The dissolution of the USSR and Yugoslavia resulted in the creation of 20 new Member States. The transition from centrally-planned to market economies in those countries, with a desire for fundamental socioeconomic changes, stimulated a search for new forms of organization, financing and service provision in the health sector.

In most of the eastern part of the region the economic situation has become very critical, with serious implications for health care. In 3 countries, for example, health personnel were not paid for six months. Armed conflicts continue to rage in 9 countries. Infectious diseases are on the rise. Polio incidence has continued to decline, however, in spite of sometimes reduced coverage. A diphtheria epidemic is in progress – with some 45 000 cases registered in 9 countries in 1994. Cholera affected 27 countries.

WHO action during the year centred on humanitarian assistance to countries affected by armed conflicts; promotion of the health-for-all policy; improvement of health care; encouragement of healthy lifestyles; and strengthening of environmental health.

Humanitarian assistance has been directed particularly to countries of former Yugoslavia, with funding from voluntary contributions. Attention is given to war victims with somatic and mental health problems. Support is also given to setting up nutrition and health surveillance, guiding health care reform and planning the reconstruction of health services. Cooperation among the medical associations of countries of former Yugoslavia is fostered, and WHO has taken the lead among United Nations agencies concerned with public health and coordinates the work of NGOs. Assistance was also provided during conflicts in Armenia, Azerbaijan, Georgia and Tajikistan.

In all countries strong emphasis is placed on promoting health for all, through the region's interactive networks such as healthy cities and the health promoting schools project, now reaching 2 000 institutions. Tobacco use remains a particular concern as international tobacco companies are engaged in aggressive marketing in central and eastern Europe and former USSR.

Because of the resurgence of infectious diseases, resources have been reallocated and specific measures taken. In cooperation with the Eastern Mediterranean region, a coordinated vaccination programme involving special vaccination days was carried out in 18 countries. A consortium of three major donors and UNICEF was set up to provide vaccines for all the countries of former USSR. Finally additional resources have been made available to combat HIV/AIDS in central and eastern Europe. In general, considerable efforts have been made at resource mobilization, resulting in a trebling of voluntary contributions over the next six years.

The European health-for-all targets, revised in 1991, provided a solid policy basis for subsequent reforms. Member States have decided that WHO should concentrate on the countries in greatest need, i.e. those in central and eastern Europe and former USSR. There is broad agreement that WHO's special mandate must be to change Europe's approach to health development, through catalytic action, innovation and leadership. In an effort to do this, reforms were made in regional management, and sharper target priorities established.

South-East Asia

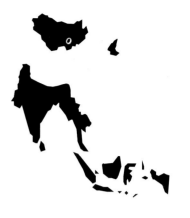

The region has a heterogeneous population amounting to a quarter of the world total. Most Member States depend on agriculture, but are increasingly turning to industrialization. Socioeconomic development plans stress improved agricultural productivity, creation of employment, upgrading of skills, greater participation of both women and men in the development process, alleviation of poverty and provision of shelter, all in a spirit of social justice and equity.

During the last decade national economies have been hurt by political uncertainty, military conflicts and natural disasters such as floods, earthquakes and drought. Instability in the Middle East and rising oil prices have also had adverse effects. In spite of this, four of the largest countries in the region have recorded satisfactory economic growth. The region accounts for almost half of the world's poor, despite efforts to curb rapid population growth which is a primary contributing factor. There are a multitude of environmental health hazards such as contaminated drinking-water, industrial and agricultural waste, air pollution, noise and pesticide poisoning.

There has been by a slow decline in mortality generally. The incidence of low birth weight is decreasing, with some countries reaching the global target of at least 90% of newborns weighing no less than 2.5 kg. Women's health is a matter of serious concern, especially in Bangladesh, Bhutan, India and Nepal.

Respiratory diseases, diseases of the digestive system, malaria, tetanus, diphtheria, tuberculosis and leprosy are the major causes of illness and death. The number of reported polio cases fell from 9 150 in 1992 to 4 520 in 1993. The Democratic People's Republic of Korea and Maldives have not reported any cases in the last four years. More recently cardiovascular diseases, cancer and other noncommunicable diseases have begun to rank as major causes of death in countries with the highest life expectancies, such as the Democratic People's Republic of Korea, Sri Lanka and Thailand.

Primary health care as the key approach to health development has been fully understood and accepted by all Member States, and substantial progress has been made in developing health care systems. However, curative care still predominates. Health workers at the first level are not adequately trained and some supervisors lack skills and motivation. A number of countries are launching administrative and organizational reforms in order to facilitate decentralization and local planning and encourage involvement and mobilization of communities in health development. Substantial progress is being made in health education of the public in the face of severe constraints such as low literacy levels, poor outreach of media and low status of women. Member States have agreed that no single country can stand alone in dealing with health problems such as HIV/AIDS, and have underlined the importance of common approaches and increased regional cooperation.

Bangladesh	Maldives
Bhutan	Mongolia
Democratic People's Republic of Korea	Myanmar
	Nepal
India	Sri Lanka
Indonesia	Thailand

Western Pacific

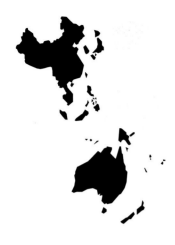

Australia
Brunei Darussalam
Cambodia
China
Cook Islands
Fiji
Japan
Kiribati
Lao People's Democratic
  Republic
Malaysia
Marshall Islands
Micronesia (Federated
  States of)
Nauru

New Zealand
Niue
Papua New Guinea
Philippines
Republic of Korea
Samoa
Singapore
Solomon Islands
Tonga
Tuvalu
Vanuatu
Viet Nam

Associate Member:
Tokelau

The Western Pacific region has 25 Member countries, with a total population of more than 1.5 billion. The region is remarkable for its heterogeneity: one country has 1.2 billion inhabitants and is the most populated in the world – others are small atolls with only 2 000 inhabitants. Some produce goods and services for nearly every country in the world – others depend to a large extent on external support.

Basically the political situation is stable, with growing collaboration among countries that have common goals. The region as a whole is characterized by continuing economic growth, although this is rarely accompanied by structural adjustments to correct imbalances in income distribution. The most significant features of demographic change are urbanization, aging and overall population growth. Rapid economic and social development has allowed the building of a comprehensive basic infrastructure and the attainment of relatively high educational levels.

Countries can be grouped in three clusters according to main causes of death. In the developed countries lifestyle-associated conditions such as cardiovascular disease, stroke, cancer and accidents predominate. The gap between these and infectious diseases is rapidly narrowing in a second group of countries. In a third group communicable diseases and malnutrition prevail, associated with severe economic difficulties. Virtually all Member States, however, report a rise in the prevalence of noncommunicable diseases.

The region has six priority areas for action: development of human resources for health; environmental health; eradication and control of selected diseases; exchange of information and experience; health promotion; and strengthening of management.

The national immunization days held in Cambodia, China, Lao People's Democratic Republic, Philippines and Viet Nam are recent examples of multisectoral and multidisciplinary approaches to mobilize different segments of society for common action. In December 1993 China carried out the largest-ever immunization campaign, reaching over 100 million children in a single day. Success has been achieved in the eradication of poliomyelitis, with the number of confirmed new cases falling to approximately 1 150 in 1993, compared with 5 963 in 1990. Prospects of having zero cases in the region by the end of 1995 are good. Progress towards the elimination of leprosy as a public health problem is likewise encouraging. Malaria continues to be a major problem for 9 countries, 8 of which have produced comprehensive plans of action. HIV/AIDS is emerging as a major health concern in the region.

In general, knowledge is available to prevent or cure many health problems, but much still remains to be done to ensure that it is used to good effect. Countries in the region are developing rapidly but economic progress in itself does not necessarily lead to improved health. A document, "New horizons in health", has been produced providing a blueprint for health development that shifts public health thinking away from emphasis on illness towards concern for underlying risk factors and conditions conducive to health.

Chapter 3
Charting the future

Trends in health

By the end of the 20th century, we could be living in a world without poliomyelitis, a world without new cases of leprosy, a world without deaths from neonatal tetanus and measles, a world without dracunculiasis (guinea-worm disease).

- Measles killed nearly 1.2 million children in 1993 and infected more than 45 million.
- Poliomyelitis killed 5 500 children in 1993 and as of that year 10 million people were disabled.
- Leprosy killed 2 400 people in 1993 and infected 600 000.
- Neonatal tetanus killed 560 000 newborn babies in 1993.
- Dracunculiasis infected 2 million people in 1993.

In these categories alone the tangible prospect is the saving of more than one and a half million children's lives. But that is not all. By the end of the century maternal mortality could be half what it was in 1993, when more than 500 000 women died in childbirth.

The world at the end of the century could be one in which infant mortality rates are no higher than 50 per 1 000 live births. At least 70 countries had higher rates than this in 1993.

In just six years mortality of children under age 5 could be no more than 70 per 1 000. At least 60 countries had higher rates than this in 1992.

We could be living in a world where less than 10% of babies are born with low birth weight. In 1990, 17% of babies were born with low birth weight. For babies born at the beginning of the 21st century, life expectancy could be at least 60 years in every country of the world. In 1993, 50 countries were below this target.

In the year 2000 we could be living in a world where at least 85% of the population will be within one hour's distance of medical care. In 1993, about 1 billion people had no access to local health services within a one-hour journey.

We could be living in a world where deaths from malaria will be cut by a fifth in at least 75% of affected countries; where the number of deaths and new infections from tuberculosis will be substantially reduced; where the number of new carriers of hepatitis B will fall by 80% as a result of childhood immunization; where deaths from heart disease in people under age 65 will be reduced by at least 15%; and where all pregnant women will have proper care.

The year 2000 could see a world where malnutrition in children under age 5 will fall by 50%; where micronutrient deficiencies from vitamin A and iodine will be eliminated; where the prevalence of iron deficiency anaemia in women of childbearing age will be reduced by 33%; and where 85% of the population will have access to safe drinking-water and 75% to sanitary facilities.

These are neither utopian targets nor naïve wishes for a perfect world. They are achievable goals – provided the world cares enough and the necessary resources are made available (*Box 16*).

Such grounds as there are for optimism about what can be achieved have to be tempered by a realistic assessment of the current situation. There have been worldwide improvements in health status and in access to health care, but not all have benefited equally. Development has not always advanced health

The year 2000 could see a world where malnutrition in children under age 5 will fall by 50%.

or quality of life. Although appropriate technologies have been devised to prevent or solve many of the major health problems facing countries, these have rarely been available to those who need them most.

Recognition of the importance of lifestyles and a healthy environment calls for greater attention to health promotion and protection, not just care. A louder voice must be given to the health consumer, the patient, with much closer collaboration between those who receive care and those who provide it. Much more attention must be paid to

Box 16. Progress towards health for all by the year 2000

Estimated global values for selected indicators related to targets of WHO's Ninth General Programme of Work (1996–2001) in 1980, 1990 and 2000 (estimates)[a]

Indicator	1980	1990	2000 (estimates)	Targets
Health status				
Life expectancy at birth (in years)				
• Global figure	61	64	67	
• (Number of countries reporting a figure of 60 years or over)	(86)	(103)	(111)	In all countries, life expectancy at birth will be 60 years or over
Infant mortality (per 1 000 live births)				
• Global figure	82	65	54	
• (Number of countries reporting a figure of 50 per 1 000 live births or under)	(70)	(83)	(99)	In all countries, infant mortality will be 50 per 1 000 live births or under
Mortality under 5 years per 1 000 live births	117	92	74	
Disease status				
Poliomyelitis incidence	630 000	116 000	nil	Eradication of poliomyelitis
Dracunculiasis prevalence (adults)	12 million	3.0 million	nil	Eradication of dracunculiasis
Leprosy prevalence	10.5 million	5.5 million	300 000	Elimination of leprosy
Neonatal tetanus incidence	1 million	0.5 million	negligible	Elimination of neonatal tetanus
Hepatitis B carriers among children	NA	350 million	400 million	Control of hepatitis B
Tuberculosis deaths	2.9 million	2.9 million	3.5 million	Control of tuberculosis
Malaria deaths	1.45 million	2.25 million	1.95 million	Control of malaria
Health care coverage (%)				
DPT (third dose)	8	83	98.5	
Poliovirus vaccine (third dose)	8	85	99	
Safe water	52	75	86	Primary health care available to whole population
Sanitation	24	71	92	
Delivery of babies by trained personnel	NA	55	60	
Health resources[b]				
Percentage of GNP expended on health	3.2	3.0		
Per capital health expenditure (in US$)	111	135		

[a] Based on data available in 1992.
[b] Central government expenditure only.
NA = not applicable; DPT = diphtheria/pertussis/tetanus vaccine; GNP = gross national product.

understanding the determinants of health, to ensuring equity in health care and services, and to improving the quality of life.

All this has to be done knowing that substantial increases in the resources allocated to health are unlikely to be forthcoming at either national or international level. Whatever resources are made available have therefore to be used judiciously to meet high-priority public health needs, whether in developed or developing countries.

Health prognosis

While the world at the end of the century may have cause to congratulate itself on advances made in improving human health, there is also a likelihood it will have to rebuke itself for opportunities missed and problems left untackled.

Technology and human determination will, it is to be hoped, have made significant inroads into certain infectious diseases. Apart from advances against poliomyelitis, measles, leprosy, neonatal tetanus, dracunculiasis and micronutrient deficiencies, the development of new vaccines could allow significant progress in the control of malaria, schistosomiasis, dengue and leishmaniasis as well as various forms of diarrhoea. The first such preparation, hepatitis B vaccine produced by DNA technology using genetically altered yeast, is now in widespread international use. The confident prediction is that more vaccines against bacterial and parasitic diseases are likely to be developed in the near future using DNA technology rather than conventional means. New insecticides are likely to be available to control the vectors of many diseases, and it is possible that genetic manipulations may be ready for application against some insect carriers.

At the moment it is difficult to be anything other than pessimistic about the spread of HIV/AIDS. The potential for an explosive spread of the virus throughout the world is truly alarming. It could undermine the great hopes for world prosperity that the emerging global economic recovery promises. Large-scale vaccine trials against HIV will begin in the near future, but there is considerable scientific uncertainty about their effectiveness; other protective measures must therefore be stressed, such as sexual abstinence, mutual monogamy with an uninfected partner and the use of condoms and other barrier methods. An effective, cheap viricide, easily usable by women, would be a highly valuable additional weapon. The need for provision of safe blood and clean needles to injecting drug users must be addressed. In addition, the continuing prejudice against those with the illness must be fought.

The global situation regarding non-communicable diseases, particularly heart disease and cancer, is difficult to predict. In the developed world rates of heart disease are falling, albeit slowly and from very high levels in some countries. Health promotion messages about the importance of diets low in fat and high in fruit and vegetables, more physical exercise and smoking cessation are all contributing to this fall.

Although in 1993 circulatory diseases accounted for only 11% of deaths in developing countries, the absolute number of those killed was more than 4.2 million. In developed countries deaths stood at 5.4 million, accounting for 47% of all mortality. Deaths from heart disease in developing countries could be expected soon to outstrip those in developed countries with the adoption of Western-style diets, smoking and sedentary lifestyles, and inadequate screening services to identify risk factors such as high blood pressure. However, recent studies of adults in the developing world indicate a major decline in cardiovascular disease mortality in women and possibly men. Such a decline is perplexing and contrary to some widely-held beliefs. Perhaps as overall mortality declines, socioeconomic improvements bring a decrease in some unknown critical risk factors, which may be of an infectious nature. If so, the declines in these unknown risk factors must be outweighing increases in

The confident prediction is that more vaccines against bacterial and parasitic diseases are likely to be developed in the near future.

smoking and other well-characterized risk factors. Alternatively, improved access to health care may be postponing deaths from cardiovascular diseases and possibly other noncommunicable diseases to after age 60.

It is already the case that more deaths from cancer occur in the developing world – some 3.5 million in 1993 – than in industrialized countries –

about 2.5 million in 1993. Projections suggest that by 2000 two-thirds of cancer cases, 10 million as against 5 million, will occur in the developing world. In developed countries lifestyle advice, screening services and in some cases curative therapy all have the potential to reduce mortality. In the developing world, however, the toll of cancer deaths will rise as a result of demographic increase and an aging population, together with rising smoking rates, changing lifestyles and inadequate access to protective measures such as cervical and breast screening and vaccinations against hepatitis B. Two-thirds of new cases will occur in those countries which have the least resources. However, cancer can be controlled through properly-formulated national cancer control programmes (*Box 17*).

Other lifestyle diseases are also likely to add to health costs in the developing world. This applies particularly to diabetes, of which there will be an expected 100 million cases by the year 2000.

Until the classic infectious diseases, particularly those of childhood, are brought under control and the resources devoted to them can be made available for other programmes, developing countries will increasingly face the double burden of continuing to cope with a legacy of the traditional diseases of poverty, while dealing with a growing number of lifestyle diseases. In the foreseeable future – say for the next 20 years at least – this burden will substantially increase the health funding needs of the least developed countries.

Priorities for the future

Achieving the goals and targets given in WHO's Ninth General Programme of Work (1996 – 2001) will be much easier if the world community that approved them can also ensure provision of the resources needed to make them a reality. Many countries are already near the targets or have long since exceeded them. In certain areas of public health cost-effective technologies exist, intervention strategies have proved effective, and organizational and managerial ex-

---

Box 17. Cancer is controllable

The present annual incidence of 9 million new cancer cases a year will increase to 15 million by 2015 according to present estimates. Two-thirds of the cases will occur in developing countries.

The science of cancer control now enables us to prevent at least a third of all cancers. Another third can be cured if diagnosed in time. For the remaining group, the incurable, palliative care exists which allows the patient the best possible quality of life. Unfortunately many countries lack suitable mechanisms to apply research findings and use available resources in a rational manner.

Regrettably countries are spending up to 90% of already scarce resources on therapies of marginal effectiveness, because the disease is diagnosed too late. Yet experience has shown that even in developing countries, which dispose of only a fraction of the total resources available, cancer control can work. For instance when women have been informed about the early symptoms of the disease, they come earlier to see health workers, who can diagnose most cases using relatively uncomplicated methods. Through this approach the proportion of cases diagnosed at an early stage, when treatment is usually successful, has risen considerably and the proportion of patients diagnosed at a later stage, when treatment is usually ineffective, has fallen.

National cancer control programmes are the key to success. Four basic activities are essential at the outset. First, the magnitude of the cancer problem must be established, even if the figure is only an estimate in the absence of reliable data. Second, policies must be reviewed and measurable cancer control objectives set, taking into account the major involvement of nongovernmental agencies in this field. Third, different strategies must be evaluated, and the best and most realistic selected. Lastly, specific activities must be decided upon, including preventive and promotive measures such as health education and regulatory action to combat smoking. Programmes must be concentrated at district level to achieve satisfactory coverage. They must include early referral for treatment such as radiotherapy with relatively cost-effective cobalt units rather than sophisticated electronic devices, and have a strong focus on palliative care.

It is important to keep district cancer programmes under constant review to ensure the most rational use of resources. This can be done by assessing the effectiveness of different activities in terms of various indicators: primary prevention, for instance, according to the observed reduction in smoking and chewing tobacco; early referral according to the promptness of presentation of cervical, oral and breast cancers; increased cure rates according to the availability of cobalt machines and the introduction of clear policies on treatment and referral; and palliative care according to the provision of oral morphine, the education of care givers and the empowerment of families to give home care.

perience and expertise are available. The following priorities are thus identified for international health action including action by WHO.

The *first priority* for the future must be to ensure value for money by refocusing resources on those who need them most; using the available resources more efficiently; mobilizing additional resources, expertise and efforts and directing them to those countries (and population groups) where the targets have not been reached. In the process, the creation of self-help environments in which the countries can initiate and sustain development activities should also be promoted. Least developed countries, particularly those that are low-income and severely indebted (most of which are in sub-Saharan Africa), must be targeted for intensive time-limited efforts for international funding and technical support.

Pragmatic outcome-oriented measures should be taken in major areas for action such as maternal and child health with adequate family planning services; immunization coverage of infants; access to safe drinking-water and sanitation; control of malaria; improved nutrition and food safety; and innovative action-oriented school health curriculums for the promotion of healthy lifestyles, particularly as regards sexual issues and HIV/AIDS. All of these should be combined with measures to strengthen local institutions and human resource bases, thus ensuring capacity building, particularly in skills which are critical to the development process. This would enable men and women to solve their own problems and establish and sustain a process that could also ensure a brighter future for their children.

The *second priority* is directly concerned with poverty reduction. Investing in health saves money as well as lives. Poverty and ill-health are closely interrelated. While poverty prevents a person from satisfying the most basic human needs (adequate food, safe water and sanitation, and access to social services such as basic health and education), ill-health inhibits an individual's ability to work, reduces earning capacity and deepens poverty. Health is thus a fundamental ingredient of the economic and social productivity of individuals and of the community, since better health increases labour productivity and enhances quality of life. Poor health not only affects the individual – it can undermine a country's ability to export its goods, or to attract much-needed investment. Recent outbreaks of cholera in Peru and plague in India did far more damage in economic terms than the numbers of people affected warranted, because of a distorted perception of the severity of the problem. Improving health is thus a social investment that contributes to greater national and global stability.

While human capital formation and investment in people are key determinants in achieving socially sustainable economic growth, the major emphasis for poverty alleviation should be on providing opportunities for people to earn their way out of their difficulties. This is possible only through increased labour productivity. Many studies have shown that low-productivity employment rather than unemployment is a major problem in developing countries. For people to be employed they must be healthy, educated and skilled; better health contributes significantly to higher productivity and thus to more earnings.

In addition to meeting basic minimum needs (e.g. access to health services, housing, education, etc.), efforts should be made to address the long-term needs of the labour market for higher productivity, which can be achieved if the workforce is healthy. This should in turn lead to a "virtuous" circle of better health, economic growth, poverty alleviation, improved welfare, and ultimately reduced social disparities, from a vicious circle of ill-health, low productivity, poverty and misery.

Poverty should thus be tackled on two fronts: one to ensure that the poor have access to primary health care (especially families with young children and vulnerable groups such as the elderly); the other to enhance the health potential of the current workforce and future workforce (schoolchildren).

Poverty reduction need not be a long-term process. Many developing countries have demonstrated that the worst forms of poverty can be rapidly reduced or eliminated.

Poverty reduction need not be a long-term process. Many developing countries have demonstrated that the worst forms of poverty can be rapidly reduced or eliminated in a relatively short time with determined, well-designed and efficiently implemented strategies.

In addition to the economic aspect there is another side to poverty – social discrimination and low status of some population groups, particularly women. Apart from economic considerations, it is essential that the social status of women be improved – this disempowerment of half of the planet must end. Women play a key role in health care, yet their own health is being jeopardized daily. The potential contributions of women to world development and improvement of the human condition are being wilfully squandered. The world can no longer afford to waste so precious a resource of potential benefit to communities and health services.

Integrating health and human development in overall public policies as outlined in WHO's Ninth General Programme of Work is a strategic move to enforce a "health in development outlook" in investment decisions at national and international levels for achieving and sustaining better health and thus ensuring a better quality of life in the future.

The **third priority** relates to public health policy. During the decade of the 1990s national and international policies have been influenced not only by the health-for-all movement but also by political and economic changes in countries and in the world at large. In a democratic setting, for instance, health and other measures require popular support. Moreover, distortions cannot be concealed; they must be corrected.

In the future it will therefore not be possible to dissociate public health policy from the overall political and economic setting. If the world community endorses the concept of equity in health, it will commit itself to achieving a better quality of life for all people, and reducing differences in health status among countries and population groups.

To put this commitment into practice, however, society must first be clear about the meaning of "equity" in the health sphere. Does it refer to "equity in health", meaning that the health status of all communities should be more or less the same? This concept of equity does take account of the individual but as a member of a community and obviously, for biological reasons, it does not imply that each person will enjoy the same level of health. Or are we talking about "equity of access to health care", meaning that every individual should have equal access to health services irrespective of the need for and outcome of use of the services?

The distinction, in essence, is between fairness in the *outcome* of health care and fairness in the *provision* of health care. These concepts are not mutually exclusive nor is the distinction always clear-cut; they do, however, reflect different perceptions of fairness. Ensuring equal access, a traditional goal of public health authorities, is essentially a matter of equitable distribution of resources. But recent studies have shown that even when access is being made equal, it has not always resulted in a significant reduction in gaps in health status within a given society or between societies. Ensuring true equity in health, which is the philosophy of health for all, calls for a far broader approach.

To remove inequities in health status, public health strategies must be outcome-oriented and take into account the changing picture of health in the world. The term "health transition" has been coined to refer to the combined effect of demographic change – in terms of fertility and mortality patterns – and epidemiological change – in terms of the growing incidence of noncommunicable diseases such as cardiovascular diseases and cancer, accidents, suicide, violence and the harmful effects of alcohol and drug use. As developing countries go through the health transition, they experience a double burden of ill-health which is determined by behaviour and the environment, as well as by biological and genetic factors.

Women play a key role in health care, yet their own health is being jeopardized daily.

Thus health status increasingly depends on social and economic circumstances over which the conventional health care sector has little control. In other words the availability and use of health care will not in themselves guarantee better health to the extent that disease is influenced by such factors as lifestyle and the working and living environment. The impact of these determinants naturally varies widely, and as a result many countries are now experiencing an "epidemiological polarization" of health i.e. persistence (and in some cases widening) of differences in disease patterns within countries. Communicable diseases are more prevalent among the poorer and rural people while middle- and upper-income urban dwellers experience more the noncommunicable diseases and conditions.

Any further improvements in health will thus call for integrated, comprehensive action addressing all the determinants of ill-health. Countries, particularly in the developing world, can no longer afford to deal with the two problems of communicable and noncommunicable diseases sequentially as in the past; they must address them simultaneously. Action is first needed within the health sector, which in turn must make intensified efforts to mobilize support from other sectors such as education, agriculture and the environment. Such a policy has financial, organizational and managerial implications.

Health professionals will inevitably be at the centre of change in the health arena. In addition to basic and specialized training, they must be given managerial skills through transdisciplinary arrangements, and be taught to address the broader problems of society. Emphasis in training must shift from the traditional recourse to technology to provide the best possible care to the individual (which in some instances may be at the expense of the community) to a concern for overall fairness and social well-being. The needs of the individual will have to be balanced with those of the community in selecting the most appro-priate technologies and making them a part of an outcome-oriented health care system. Within that framework health services must be provided pragmatically in a way that gives each individual access to an entry-point of essential health care from which it is possible for them to seek other relevant services as and when needed.

Ethical considerations will figure prominently in the health care of the future in the broad sense of ensuring equity in health outcome and the specific sense of addressing such questions as new reproductive health technology, medical research, human genome studies and the allocation of scarce resources. In this situation, advocacy and technical support will be expected not only in establishing international health standards but in designing blueprints for action.

Finally, the *fourth priority* relates to strengthening national capabilities for emergency relief and humanitarian assistance in the health sector. The new policy of "emergency management for sustainable development" will provide a bridge between relief work and development proper, the aim being to provide a long-term solution for reducing human suffering and avoiding economic loss due to epidemics, complex emergencies and mass population displacements.

The health problems of the future are awesome. But the situation is not hopeless, and much can be done to tackle them with the knowledge we already possess. To succeed, the world will have to care more and to try harder. Martin Luther King, referring to the civil rights struggle in the United States in the 1960s, once wrote: "We shall have to repent in this generation, not so much for the evil deeds of wicked people, but for the appalling silence of the good people".

Today, as a new generation approaches a new century, it is time for the appalling silence over health inequities in the world to be broken – and for the cries for help of hundreds of millions of people to be heard.

It is time for the appalling silence over health inequities in the world to be broken.

The evolution of WHO

In 1948 the scars of the second world war had barely begun to heal. Massive recovery and reconstruction activities were being launched in Europe and Japan. The colonial era was coming to an end, and many countries were in the process of liberation. Added to the huge numbers of people killed or disabled during the war, millions were dying from preventable diseases. In the world community's cautious quest for new international relationships that might lead to a better future, improving the health of humanity emerged as a common bond.

The First World Health Assembly, in June 1948, approved a programme of work that listed its top priorities in the following order: malaria, maternal and child health, tuberculosis, venereal diseases, nutrition and environmental sanitation.

Today, 47 years later, in spite of significant improvements in human health, particularly in terms of mortality reduction, great burdens of suffering and disease are still with us. Half a century of lessons learned in eradicating and controlling diseases, expanding health care coverage and making the best use of available resources have guided the world community, including WHO, on the way to further progress. This special chapter presents a review of international health and the evolution of WHO.

Ancient scourges in a modern world

Measured against the life span of diseases that have plagued the world throughout recorded history, WHO today is still in its early infancy. In Ancient Egypt as long ago as 3000 BC, diseases such as tuberculosis, poliomyelitis and syphilis were rampant. Leprosy is at least as ancient. Researchers have found traces in Egyptian mummies of schistosomiasis, a parasitic waterborne disease. Today that same disease affects some 200 million people.

Smallpox and measles were recognized in Asia at least 1 000 years ago. In the course of some 30 years during the 14th century bubonic plague killed perhaps as many as a quarter of the population of Europe, leading to the introduction by the city state of Venice of the first systematic quarantine regulations.

The eradication of smallpox in the late 1970s is regarded as one of WHO's greatest achievements, and measles has been eliminated from much of the industrialized world. But plague, as the outbreak in India in 1994 vividly illustrated, still persists in a number of countries with well-known natural foci. Close and continuous surveillance of this and other major diseases is today an important part of the International Health Regulations.

The cholera pandemic which invaded Europe in 1830 from India through Russia caused death on a massive scale. This, together with the tolls inflicted by plague and yellow fever, prompted in the late 1840s a greater recognition among affected countries of the need for international collaboration to prevent disease, essentially through the quarantine approach. One hundred years later the establishment of WHO was a major step towards fulfilling that need.

There were other important steps along the way. In 1864 the Red Cross, the first international humanitarian

The eradication of smallpox in the late 1970s is regarded as one of WHO's greatest achievements, and measles has been eliminated from much of the industrialized world.

agency, was founded with the aim of giving emergency aid to the wounded of wars without choosing sides. The rapid expansion of scientific knowledge and the consequent need to coordinate research and exchange information prompted the establishment of the Pan American Sanitary Bureau in 1902, and the *Bureau international d'Hygiène publique* (OIHP) in 1907. In 1920 a constitution was drafted for a new health organization under the League of Nations, itself formed as a consequence of the first world war. This health organization collaborated closely with OIHP for many years, collecting and distributing epidemiological information, until the second world war prevented their continued functioning.

When the war ended, the majority of the world's population were still living in extreme poverty and suffering from chronic malnutrition, communicable diseases and parasitic infections to name a few. Children were at particularly high risk. Many of the existing health services, for instance in cities in Europe, northern Africa and Asia, had been severely disrupted. Structured health services were in any case rare, and where they did exist huge segments of the population – usually the most vulnerable people who could not pay for the often questionable care that was available – were excluded.

The need for a world health organization

Against this background the imperative need was recognized for a new world body capable of grouping resources for health, setting health goals and providing a forum for the exchange of health information and experience. But in the immediate postwar years no international health agency could do other than make an all-out effort to alleviate the epidemics that were sweeping the war-ravaged developed countries, colonial territories and some newly independent nations.

There were some models of national health services, usually based on the principle of compulsory health insur-

ance, with the state taking responsibility for the poorest people, and individuals contributing according to their means. But it soon became clear that such models would not work in countries where virtually no medical treatment was available, where trained health workers were scarce, and where most people would never be able to make the financial contributions required to support health services. A crucial task of a new body would therefore be to help countries build up or reconstruct broadly-based health services and see how best to organize them so as to bring health care to the people.

An international conference in San Francisco in 1945 drew up guidelines for the functioning of the United Nations. During those discussions emerged the memorable statement attributed to the United States archbishop, later Cardinal Spellman, that "medicine is one of the pillars of peace". The United Nations set up a technical preparatory committee to establish the specialized agency that would emerge as WHO. An international health conference in June 1946 was dominated by new aspirations for a better world and better health for the peoples of the world.

In a message read to the conference on his behalf, United States President Harry S. Truman said: "Modern transportation has made it impossible for a nation to protect itself against the introduction of disease by quarantine. This makes it necessary to develop strong health services in every country which must be coordinated through international action. The new health organization will serve in this field. Just as international cooperation in science played a most important part in winning the war, so will such cooperation win the battle against disease and malnutrition".

The conference agreed that the new body would be known as the World Health Organization and produced a constitution for it, specifying that its role would be to act as the directing and coordinating authority in international health, giving assistance to governments on request. People and their right to

The United Nations set up a technical preparatory committee to establish the specialized agency that would emerge as WHO. An international health conference in June 1946 was dominated by new aspirations for a better world and better health for the peoples of the world.

health were to be at the centre of the development process. International solidarity in the fight for health would replace the basically quarantine-inspired approach of earlier international health initiatives. WHO now comprises six regions (see *Map 7*).

The First World Health Assembly in 1948 was attended by 53 delegates from WHO's 55 Member States, the majority in the industrialized world. Its top priorities are listed at the beginning of this chapter, but there was some emphasis too on the socioeconomic, cultural and political dimensions of health. The main stress, however, was on the control of disease, and WHO's first two decades were dominated by mass campaigns in country after country against tuberculosis, malaria, yaws, syphilis, smallpox and leprosy, among others.

Declaring war on disease: victories and defeats

At the beginning of the 1950s there were believed to be around 20 million cases worldwide of yaws, a tropical disease mainly affecting the skin and bones. A single injection of penicillin was enough to cure it. Between 1950 when the first yaws campaign was launched in Haiti and 1965, a total of 46 million patients in 49 countries were successfully treated, and the disease was no longer a significant public health problem in most of the developing world. But the success of the campaign was misleading. It created an ill-founded optimism among health workers that other diseases could be controlled as easily.

In 1951 WHO took on the responsibility of coordinating a worldwide tuberculosis campaign largely funded by UNICEF. Initially the campaign concentrated on vaccinating children with BCG. By 1960 serious doubts about the campaign approach began to surface. The campaign was operating in an indiscriminate manner, achieving high coverage in regions where prevalence of the disease was low, and failing to reach populations whose chances of contracting the disease were high. Voices were

therefore raised in favour of integrating BCG vaccination with other preventive and curative components of health services.

Also in 1951 WHO teams were at work in 22 malaria control projects, mostly in Asia, again with huge support from UNICEF. Malaria had been identified as the world's gravest threat to public health. The initial results were extremely encouraging. By 1955 the number of cases worldwide had dropped by at least one-third. The Health Assembly that year urged Member States to abandon malaria control and make eradication of the disease a priority of the highest order and urgency. But by 1966 the situation looked much less promising. Although 60% of the population of the originally malarious regions of the world were now living in areas where the disease had been eradicated or was no longer a major health problem, there were innumerable setbacks. In Africa virtually no progress had been made. Poorly developed health services were unable to cope, and in many countries the cost of antimalarial efforts was unbearable. In 1970 the Health Assembly recognized that malaria eradication was generally impracticable, and called instead for malaria control programmes to be reintroduced. Today WHO still gives high priority to the battle against the disease. But there is now a sense of realism about what can be achieved, especially in Africa, where improvements in economic and social conditions and in access to primary health care have been slow; 1970 was thus a turning point in the malaria battle.

1966 saw the opening of a new front, this time against smallpox. Against a background of widespread disenchantment with mass campaigns against a single disease, the Health Assembly nevertheless voted to make an all-out effort to eradicate smallpox within the next 10 years. At that time smallpox victims were estimated to number 10-15 million a year worldwide, of whom 1.5-2 million died. The disease was endemic in 30 countries. Eradication of smallpox was made possible by a combination of factors. There were no

WHO's first two decades were dominated by mass campaigns in country after country against tuberculosis, malaria, yaws, syphilis, smallpox and leprosy, among others.

known animal reservoirs, and no long-term carriers of the smallpox virus. Patients who recovered had essentially life-long immunity. People with subclinical infections did not transmit the disease. Case detection was relatively simple. Above all a highly effective, stable and easily administered vaccine that conferred long-term protection was available. The smallpox campaign was the first global effort that has succeeded in eradicating a major disease. The achievement of this goal was certified in May 1980.

Box 18. Primary Health Care

In 1978, the International Conference on Primary Health Care held in Alma-Ata identified the following eight essential elements of primary health care:

■ education concerning prevailing health problems and methods for addressing them

■ promotion of food supply and proper nutrition

■ provision of an adequate supply of safe water and basic sanitation

■ maternal and child health care, including family planning

■ immunization against the major infectious diseases

■ prevention and control of locally endemic diseases

■ appropriate treatment of common diseases and injuries

■ provision of essential drugs.

Immunization programmes

The mass campaigns against single diseases of the first decades gave way to WHO's Expanded Programme on Immunization aimed at protecting by the year 2000 all children against six vaccine-preventable diseases – measles, diphtheria, pertussis, tetanus, poliomyelitis and tuberculosis – in their first year of life. Global coverage with the vaccines reached its peak at the end of 1990 when the goal of immunizing 80% of all children by the age of 1 year was achieved. The main factors inhibiting further progress have been insufficient political commitment by countries, civil unrest, donor fatigue and lack of resources.

After smallpox the next vaccine-preventable disease targeted for eradication is poliomyelitis. In 1992 no cases were reported in the western hemisphere. By maintaining surveillance in the poliomyelitis-free areas and intensifying control measures elsewhere, WHO expects the disease to be eradicated by the year 2000.

In 1994 WHO established a global programme for vaccines and immunization aimed at coordinating all activities in this field carried out within the Organization and by other agencies. The programme is also responsible for WHO's contribution to the multiagency children's vaccine initiative, launched in 1990 to stimulate the provision of improved, safe, reliable and affordable vaccines for the developing world and which can be given in a single procedure. The long-term goal is to achieve a world where all people at risk are protected against vaccine-preventable diseases.

Health for all by the year 2000

Ever since its inception WHO has pursued as its overriding goal the achievement of better health for all people everywhere, in the sense not simply of survival, but of enhanced quality of life. Yet a review in the early 1970s showed that more than half the population of the globe did not have access to adequate health care. The gap between developed and developing countries in levels of health was widening. Gaps were also evident between different groups of populations within countries.

In 1977 the Health Assembly resolved that the main social target for governments and WHO in the coming decades should be "the attainment by all citizens of the world by the year 2000 of a level of health that will permit them to lead a socially and economically productive life".

In September 1978 delegates from 134 countries and 67 United Nations bodies and nongovernmental organizations met at Alma-Ata (Kazakhstan) for an international conference on primary health care. This led to the Declaration of Alma-Ata, unanimously endorsed by the Health Assembly in 1979. Every one of WHO's Member States was now committed to a form of public health action that implied fundamental changes in the distribution and use of resources and in the responsibilities within the health care system, government and society.

The declaration, a landmark document in the history of international health, stated that primary health care was to be the key to attaining the target of health for all by the year 2000 as part of overall development and in the spirit of human justice. It called on all governments to formulate national policies, strategies and plans of action to launch and sustain primary health care as part of a comprehensive national health system and in coordination with other sectors (*Box 18*).

In 1981 the Health Assembly approved the definitive global strategy for health for all by the year 2000. Global targets for health were established for the year 2000, and have since been the criteria against which all health development efforts have been measured. At a conference in Riga in 1988, attended by ministers of health, finance and planning, it was noted that primary health care coverage had greatly improved in many countries, but that there were still many deficiencies.

WHO sets the standards

The establishment of standards in such fields as vaccines, drugs and laboratory tests has been a permanent part of WHO's work. These instruments have been universally accepted as representing the best available technical advice of the moment and have been the basis for the Organization's reputation as the undisputed authority in health matters.

In pursuance of WHO's constitutional functions in regard to the standardization particularly of biological and pharmaceutical products, the WHO Expert Committee on Biological Standardization has been meeting every year since 1951 to formulate standards which

are recognized worldwide. They enable drug and vaccine manufacturers to ensure the availability of safe and efficacious biologicals as well as standard product dosage and diagnostic tests. Because of the scientific credibility of WHO, this gives confidence to patients, doctors and other health personnel for using drugs of proven efficacy and valid diagnostic procedures.

WHO's contribution to the Codex Alimentarius Commission on food standards and the International Code of Marketing of Breast-milk Substitutes are an example of the Organization using

Box 19. *The International Classification of Diseases*

The International Statistical Classification of Diseases and Related Health Problems (ICD), under different names, has so far undergone 10 revisions. The first ICD or ICD-zero was prepared in 1893 by Jacques Bertillon of France under a mandate given to the International Statistical Institute. Subsequent revision conferences were convened by France in 1900 (ICD-1), 1909 (ICD-2), 1920 (ICD-3), 1929 (ICD-4) and 1938 (ICD-5), the latter two under the auspices of the institute and the Health Organisation of the League of Nations. The international conference for the sixth revision was convened in Paris in 1948 with the collaboration of the Interim Commission of the World Health Organization. WHO has thus been responsible for the last five revisions of the classification.

Before ICD-6 the classification was used only for mortality statistics. That revision was expanded to make it suitable for the collection of morbidity statistics. ICD-7 in 1955 was limited to essential changes and amendments of errors and inconsistencies. ICD-8 in 1965 was more radical than ICD-7, but left unchanged the basic structure of the classification and the general philosophy of classifying diseases, whenever possible, according to their etiology rather than a particular manifestation.

In 1975 ICD-9 retained the same basic structure, although with much additional detail, and introduced classifications of impairments, disabilities and handicaps (ICIDH), and of procedures in medicine as supplements. ICIDH seeks to establish, for international acceptance and use, uniform definitions and terminology – often confused and misused – in the field of rehabilitation. In the course of successive revisions ICD has thus expanded to cover the whole spectrum of health.

ICD-10, the 21st century classification, was adopted by the Health Assembly in 1990. It initiated the use of an alphanumeric coding scheme of one letter followed by three numbers at the four-character level, and constitutes the "core" of a family of disease- and health-related classifications. The purpose of the classification is to serve as a tool for comparisons between countries at the same point in time, and within and between countries over time, thus enabling the compilation of comparable statistics for decision-making in disease prevention and health care, and facilitating the collection of epidemiological data for research purposes.

its moral and technical authority to help different interest groups to reach a consensus.

Another type of standard relates to the classification of diseases (*Box 19*). The recently published tenth revision of the *International Classification of Diseases* (ICD-10) is intended to serve as a tool for facilitating the collection of epidemiological data for comparisons between countries at the same point in time, and within and between countries over time, and thus enabling the compilation of comparable statistics for decision-making in disease prevention and for research purposes.

WHO's role in health planning has changed over the years, reflecting the Organization's evolving policy on health development in general.

Human resources for health

Training physicians and raising the standards of medical schools in developing countries, helping countries organize schools for nurses and midwives and launching training courses for allied health personnel have always been an important part of WHO's work. The concept of primary health care has switched much of the emphasis to training directed towards a wide range of health care workers at community level, particularly in developing countries, rather than towards health professionals as such.

Managing health development

WHO's role in health planning has changed over the years, reflecting the Organization's evolving policy on health development in general.

Before 1965 planning was carried out as a routine function of public health administration. Between 1965 and 1970 WHO supported the development of specific concepts and methods of national health planning. The next five years saw the application of the systems approach, exploration of computer modelling and the introduction of health project planning and management.

The period 1975 to 1980 saw the advent of health sector programming (also

referred to as country health programming) and the initiation of the managerial process for national health development. Since 1990 WHO has stressed the importance of evaluation, with little attention paid to health planning as such.

Meanwhile, futures studies used in other sectors and for national planning development in some countries, began to be used in the health sector. The futures approach utilizes such methods as visioning, alternative scenario development, trend analysis and forecasting, and dynamic modelling, and may well be the basis for health planning in the 21st century.

The contribution of NGOs

The 1945 San Francisco conference which drew up the Charter of the United Nations recognized the advantages to be found in the enthusiasm, knowledge and experience of international associations, and authorized the Economic and Social Council of the UN to consult with, and make effective use of, nongovernmental organizations (NGOs). WHO's constitution goes a step further, authorizing not only consultation but cooperation with NGOs in health matters. Official relationship is granted by WHO's Executive Board to NGOs that deal with matters falling within the competence of the Organization and pursue aims and purposes in conformity with the spirit, purposes and principles of its constitution.

At the end of 1957 some 40 NGOs were in official relations with WHO. During the first years most of them dealt with a particular branch of medical science or research and represented professional groups; only a few had a more general interest in health. Nevertheless it was recognized that collaboration with these organizations was useful for obtaining information, making WHO's objectives known and stimulating interest in international health work. 1959 saw the first admission to official relations of an NGO representing persons suffering from a specific health problem, namely the World Federation of the Deaf. By January 1994 the total had reached 184 (*Annex 2*).

Being relatively unbound by the legislative and policy constraints of governments, NGOs have the flexibility to experiment with innovative and alternative approaches to solving health problems. Many can effectively mobilize large numbers of volunteers and thus play a dynamic role in national health development. Growing numbers of NGOs are becoming involved in advocacy, health promotion and technical cooperation, as well as fund-raising and provision of resources both for national health development and for WHO's technical programmes, often working closely with them. In 1990 the WHO Executive Board noted a rapid growth of NGOs and stressed that among the most important criteria for admission into official relations with WHO must be that a major part of the NGO's work is relevant to and has bearing on the achievement of health for all.

The political context

When the movement for health for all was launched, it was assumed that economic growth would continue nearly everywhere and that richer countries would give substantial assistance to the poorer nations provided their case was well presented. The global economic crisis of the late 1970s and early 1980s undermined both those assumptions. The break-up of the USSR, with the emergence of many newly independent states, the end of the cold war and the demise of communism led to more emphasis being placed on privatization, decentralization and liberalization. In turn the accompanying changes in health care systems led to new problems and distortions, and to moves for more central control of health care in some countries. Equity in health and health care, health as a human right and ethical issues became a concern in many countries.

The post-cold war period prompted hopes of a "peace dividend" from the reduction in military spending. But it failed to materialize. Instead global recession, the seemingly never-ending rise in health costs and growing expectations for health care created serious funding problems and necessitated painful cutbacks in health care, even in rich countries. As global East-West tensions subsided, armed conflicts between and within countries seemed to take on new dimensions.

WHO has learned that health cannot be divorced from politics. Until recently few political leaders believed that health was a worthwhile economic or political investment. The strategy of health for all has been endorsed at the highest political level, but a gap remains between what is preached and what is practised. In many countries the health sector wields little political power or influence in decisions about the allocation of public funds. Expenditure on health care has tended to be viewed simply as a drain on scarce resources, rather than as an investment in the nation's future.

Professional and financial interests, bureaucratic resistance to change and political considerations have been underlying reasons for the sometimes slow application of WHO guidelines; yet the Organization's position as the health technical agency and the health conscience of the world has helped to ensure acceptance of its advice over time. The eradication of smallpox was made possible by close collaboration under WHO's auspices by a great many countries without regard to political differences. WHO's advocacy of the concept of health for all has been accepted by governments worldwide.

The emphasis in public health has swung away from the technical and scientific thrust of the early disease-oriented campaigns towards understanding the underlying determinants of health, and seeking to influence them in a positive way through health promotion directed at individuals, communities and

> *The strategy of health for all has been endorsed at the highest political level, but a gap remains between what is preached and what is practised.*

governments. This unfortunately diluted traditional and effective measures such as the maintenance of adequate surveillance systems to trigger effective action for the control of communicable diseases.

The way ahead

WHO's general programmes of work, now covering periods of six years, give principles and policies for the functioning of the Organization. They also provide a framework for detailed workplans and budgeting. Over the years the programmes have responded to, and often anticipated, the major health concerns of Member countries. The ninth programme (1996-2001) fixes goals and targets for WHO's global health action. It focuses on lessening of inequities in health, control of rising costs, the eradication or elimination of selected infectious diseases, the fight against chronic diseases, and the promotion of healthy behaviour and a healthy environment.

The challenge for the future is to mobilize WHO's Member States to adopt policies and plans that will guarantee the provision of comprehensive integrated health services to each and every member of the community.

Map 7. WHO regions and the areas they serve as of December 1994

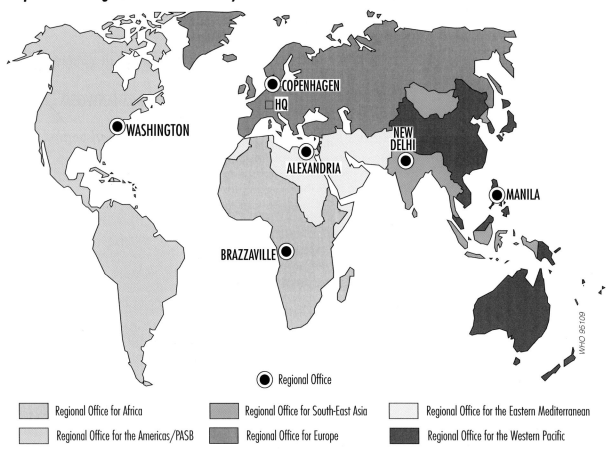

COPENHAGEN
HQ
WASHINGTON
NEW DELHI
ALEXANDRIA
MANILA
BRAZZAVILLE

● Regional Office

Regional Office for Africa	
Regional Office for the Americas/PASB	
Regional Office for South-East Asia	
Regional Office for Europe	
Regional Office for the Eastern Mediterranean	
Regional Office for the Western Pacific	

WHO 95109

Annex 1

Members and Associate Members of WHO

WHO has 189 Member States and two Associate Members. They are listed below with the date on which they became a party to the constitution or were admitted to associate membership.

Afghanistan 19 April 1948	Comoros 09 December 1975
Albania 26 May 1947	Congo 26 October 1960
Algeria* 08 November 1962	Cook Islands 09 May 1984
Angola 15 May 1976	Costa Rica 17 March 1949
Antigua and Barbuda* 12 March 1984	Côte d'Ivoire* 28 October 1960
Argentina* 22 October 1948	Croatia* 11 June 1992
Armenia 04 May 1992	Cuba* 09 May 1948
Australia* 02 February 1948	Cyprus* 16 January 1961
Austria* 30 June 1947	Czech Republic* 22 January 1993
Azerbaijan 02 October 1992	Democratic People's Republic of Korea 19 May 1973
Bahamas* 01 April 1974	Denmark* 19 April 1948
Bahrain* 02 November 1971	Djibouti 10 March 1978
Bangladesh 19 May 1972	Dominica* 13 August 1981
Barbados* 25 April 1967	Dominican Republic 21 June 1948
Belarus* 07 April 1948	Ecuador* 01 March 1949
Belgium* 25 June 1948	Egypt* 16 December 1947
Belize 23 August 1990	El Salvador 22 June 1948
Benin 20 September 1960	Equatorial Guinea 05 May 1980
Bhutan 08 March 1982	Eritrea 24 September 1993
Bolivia 23 December 1949	Estonia 31 March 1993
Bosnia and Herzegovina* 10 September 1992	Ethiopia 11 April 1947
Botswana* 26 February 1975	Fiji* 01 January 1972
Brazil* 02 June 1948	Finland* 07 October 1947
Brunei Darussalam 25 March 1985	France 16 June 1948
Bulgaria* 09 June 1948	Gabon* 21 November 1960
Burkina Faso* 04 October 1960	Gambia* 26 April 1971
Burundi 22 October 1962	Georgia 26 May 1992
Cambodia* 17 May 1950	Germany* 29 May 1951
Cameroon* 06 May 1960	Ghana* 08 April 1957
Canada 29 August 1946	Greece* 12 March 1948
Cape Verde 05 January 1976	Grenada 04 December 1974
Central African Republic* 20 September 1960	Guatemala* 26 August 1949
Chad 01 January 1961	Guinea* 19 May 1959
Chile* 15 October 1948	Guinea-Bissau 29 July 1974
China* 22 July 1946	Guyana* 27 September 1966
Colombia 14 May 1959	Haiti* 12 August 1947

* Member States that have acceded to the Convention on the Privileges and Immunities of the Specialized Agencies and its Annex VII.

Honduras   08 April 1949
Hungary*   17 June 1948
Iceland   17 June 1948
India*   12 January 1948
Indonesia*   23 May 1950
Iran (Islamic Republic of)*   23 November 1946
Iraq*   23 September 1947
Ireland*   20 October 1947
Israel   21 June 1949
Italy*   11 April 1947
Jamaica*   21 March 1963
Japan*   16 May 1951
Jordan*   07 April 1947
Kazakhstan   19 August 1992
Kenya*   27 January 1964
Kiribati   26 July 1984
Kuwait*   09 May 1960
Kyrgyzstan   29 April 1992
Lao People's Democratic Republic*   17 May 1950
Latvia   04 December 1991
Lebanon   19 January 1949
Lesotho*   07 July 1967
Liberia   14 March 1947
Libyan Arab Jamahiriya*   16 May 1952
Lithuania   25 November 1991
Luxembourg*   03 June 1949
Madagascar*   16 January 1961
Malawi*   09 April 1965
Malaysia*   24 April 1958
Maldives*   05 November 1965
Mali*   17 October 1960
Malta*   01 February 1965
Marshall Islands   05 June 1991
Mauritania   07 March 1961
Mauritius*   09 December 1968
Mexico   07 April 1948
Micronesia (Federated States of)   14 August 1991
Monaco   08 July 1948
Mongolia*   18 April 1962
Morocco*   14 May 1956
Mozambique   11 September 1975
Myanmar   01 July 1948

Namibia   23 April 1990
Nauru   09 May 1994
Nepal*   02 September 1953
Netherlands*   25 April 1947
New Zealand*   10 December 1946
Nicaragua*   24 April 1950
Niger*   05 October 1960
Nigeria*   25 November 1960
Niue   04 May 1994
Norway*   18 August 1947
Oman   28 May 1971
Pakistan*   23 June 1948
Panama   20 February 1951
Papua New Guinea   29 April 1976
Paraguay   04 January 1949
Peru   11 November 1949
Philippines*   09 July 1948
Poland*   06 May 1948
Portugal   13 February 1948
Qatar   11 May 1972
Republic of Korea*   17 August 1949
Republic of Moldova   04 May 1992
Romania*   08 June 1948
Russian Federation*   24 March 1948
Rwanda*   07 November 1962
Saint Kitts and Nevis   03 December 1984
Saint Lucia*   11 November 1980
Saint Vincent and the
    Grenadines   02 September 1983
Samoa   16 May 1962
San Marino   12 May 1980
Sao Tome and Principe   23 March 1976
Saudi Arabia   26 May 1947
Senegal*   31 October 1960
Seychelles*   11 September 1979
Sierra Leone*   20 October 1961
Singapore*   25 February 1966
Slovakia*   04 February 1993
Slovenia*   07 May 1992
Solomon Islands   04 April 1983
Somalia   26 January 1961
South Africa   07 August 1947

Spain*   28 May 1951
Sri Lanka   07 July 1948
Sudan   14 May 1956
Suriname   25 March 1976
Swaziland   16 April 1973
Sweden*   28 August 1947
Switzerland   26 March 1947
Syrian Arab Republic   18 December 1946
Tajikistan   04 May 1992
Thailand*   26 September 1947
The Former Yugoslav Republic
    of Macedonia   22 April 1993
Togo*   13 May 1960
Tonga*   14 August 1975
Trinidad and Tobago*   03 January 1963
Tunisia*   14 May 1956
Turkey   02 January 1948
Turkmenistan   02 July 1992
Tuvalu   07 May 1993
Uganda*   07 March 1963
Ukraine*   03 April 1948
United Arab Emirates   30 March 1972
United Kingdom of Great Britain
    and Northern Ireland*   22 July 1946
United Republic of Tanzania*   15 March 1962
United States of America   21 June 1948
Uruguay*   22 April 1949
Uzbekistan   22 May 1992
Vanuatu   07 March 1983
Venezuela   07 July 1948
Viet Nam   17 May 1950
Yemen   20 November 1953
Yugoslavia*   19 November 1947
Zaire*   24 February 1961
Zambia*   02 February 1965
Zimbabwe*   16 May 1980

Associate Members

Puerto Rico   07 May 1992
Tokelau   08 May 1991

* Member States that have acceded to the Convention on the
  Privileges and Immunities of the Specialized Agencies and its
  Annex VII.

Annex 2

Nongovernmental Organizations in Official Relations with WHO at 31 December 1994

African Medical and Research Foundation International

Aga Khan Foundation

Association of the Institutes and Schools of Tropical Medicine in Europe

Christoffel-Blindenmission

CMC-Churches' Action for Health

Collegium Internationale Neuro-Psychopharmacologicum

Commonwealth Association for Mental Handicap and Developmental Disabilities

Commonwealth Medical Association

Commonwealth Pharmaceutical Association

Council for International Organizations of Medical Sciences

Helen Keller International Incorporated

Industry Council for Development

Inter-American Association of Sanitary and Environmental Engineering

Inter-Parliamentary Union

International Academy of Legal Medicine

International Academy of Pathology

International Agency for the Prevention of Blindness

International Air Transport Association

International Alliance of Women

International Association for Accident and Traffic Medicine

International Association for Adolescent Health

International Association for Child and Adolescent Psychiatry and Allied Professions

International Association for Suicide Prevention

International Association for the Study of Pain

International Association for the Study of the Liver

International Association of Agricultural Medicine and Rural Health

International Association of Cancer Registries

International Association of Hydatid Disease

International Association of Lions Clubs

International Association of Logopedics and Phoniatrics

International Association of Medical Laboratory Technologists

International Association on Water Quality

International Astronautical Federation

International Bureau for Epilepsy

International Catholic Committee of Nurses and Medico-Social Assistants

International Clearinghouse for Birth Defects Monitoring Systems

International College of Surgeons

International Commission on Non-ionizing Radiation

International Commission on Occupational Health

International Commission on Radiation Units and Measurements

International Commission on Radiological Protection

International Committee of the Red Cross

International Confederation of Midwives

International Conference of Deans of French Language Faculties of Medicine

International Consultation on Urological Diseases

International Council for Control of Iodine Deficiency Disorders

International Council for Laboratory Animal Science

International Council for Standardization in Haematology

International Council of Nurses

International Council of Scientific Unions

International Council of Societies of Pathology

International Council of Women

International Council on Alcohol and Addictions

International Council on Jewish Social and Welfare Services

International Council on Social Welfare

International Cystic Fibrosis (Mucoviscidosis) Association

International Dental Federation

International Diabetes Federation

International Electrotechnical Commission

International Epidemiological Association

International Ergonomics Association

International Eye Foundation

International Federation for Family Life Promotion

International Federation for Housing and Planning

International Federation for Information Processing

International Federation for Medical and Biological Engineering

International Federation for Preventive and Social Medicine

International Federation of Business and Professional Women

International Federation of Chemical, Energy and General Workers' Unions

International Federation of Clinical Chemistry

International Federation of Fertility Societies

International Federation of Gynecology and Obstetrics

International Federation of Health Records Organizations

International Federation of Hospital Engineering

International Federation of Hydrotherapy and Climatotherapy

International Federation of Medical Students Associations

International Federation of Multiple Sclerosis Societies

International Federation of Ophthalmological Societies

International Federation of Oto-Rhino-Laryngological Societies

International Federation of Pharmaceutical Manufacturers Associations

International Federation of Physical Medicine and Rehabilitation

International Federation of Red Cross and Red Crescent Societies

International Federation of Sports Medicine

International Federation of Surgical Colleges

International Federation on Ageing

International Group of National Associations of Manufacturers of Agrochemical Products

International Hospital Federation

International Lactation Consultant Association

International League against Epilepsy

International League of Associations for Rheumatology

International League of Dermatological Societies

International Leprosy Association

International Leprosy Union

International Life Sciences Institute

International Medical Informatics Association

International Medical Society of Paraplegia

International Occupational Hygiene Association

International Organization against Trachoma

International Organization for Standardization

International Organization of Consumers Unions

International Pediatric Association

International Pharmaceutical Federation

International Physicians for the Prevention of Nuclear War

International Planned Parenthood Federation

International Radiation Protection Association

International Society and Federation of Cardiology

International Society for Biomedical Research on Alcoholism

International Society for Burn Injuries

International Society for Human and Animal Mycology

International Society for Preventive Oncology

International Society for Prosthetics and Orthotics

International Society for the Study of Behavioural Development

International Society of Biometeorology

International Society of Blood Transfusion

International Society of Chemotherapy

International Society of Hematology

International Society of Nurses in Cancer Care

International Society of Orthopaedic Surgery and Traumatology

International Society of Radiographers and Radiological Technologists

International Society of Radiology

International Society of Surgery

International Sociological Association

International Solid Wastes and Public Cleansing Association

International Special Dietary Foods Industries

International Union against Cancer

International Union against Tuberculosis and Lung Disease

International Union against the Venereal Diseases and the Treponematoses

International Union for Conservation of Nature and Natural Resources

International Union for Health Promotion and Education

International Union of Architects

International Union of Biological Sciences

International Union of Family Organizations

International Union of Immunological Societies

International Union of Local Authorities

International Union of Microbiological Societies

International Union of Nutritional Sciences

International Union of Pharmacology

International Union of Pure and Applied Chemistry

International Union of Toxicology

International Water Supply Association

Joint Commission on International Aspects of Mental Retardation

La Leche League International

Medical Women's International Association

Medicus Mundi Internationalis (International Organization for Cooperation in Health Care)

Mother and Child International

National Council for International Health

Network of Community-Oriented Educational Institutions for Health Sciences

OXFAM

Rehabilitation International

Rotary International

Save the Children Fund (UK)

Soroptimist International

The Population Council

The Royal Commonwealth Society for the Blind (Sight Savers)

World Assembly of Youth

World Association for Psychosocial Rehabilitation

World Association of Girl Guides and Girl Scouts

World Association of Societies of (Anatomic and Clinical) Pathology

World Association of the Major Metropolises

World Blind Union

World Confederation for Physical Therapy

World Federation for Medical Education

World Federation for Mental Health

World Federation of Associations of Poisons Centres and Clinical Toxicology Centres

World Federation of Hemophilia

World Federation of Neurology

World Federation of Neurosurgical Societies

World Federation of Nuclear Medicine and Biology

World Federation of Occupational Therapists

World Federation of Parasitologists

World Federation of Proprietary Medicine Manufacturers

World Federation of Public Health Associations

World Federation of Societies of Anaesthesiologists

World Federation of the Deaf

World Federation of United Nations Associations

World Hypertension League

World Medical Association

World Organization of Family Doctors

World Organization of the Scout Movement

World Psychiatric Association

World Rehabilitation Fund

World Veterans Federation

World Veterinary Association

World Vision International

Annex 3
Statistics

Explanatory notes

The World Health Report 1995 – Bridging the gaps presents an overview of the global health situation based on an assessment carried out in 1994 using 1993 data. The content of the report was determined essentially by the availability of information concerning key health and health-related indicators. However, the majority of Member States still experience great difficulty in obtaining valid and timely data on many indicators. Official statistics reported to WHO were incomplete, often not comparable among countries, nor up to date. It was often necessary to supplement data from national reports and publications with reasonably reliable estimates for one or more indicators. Considerable efforts were made to assemble and validate the best available and reasonably reliable data from such sources as reports on monitoring progress towards health for all by the year 2000, WHO regional offices, WHO technical programmes and WHO collaborating centres. Reference was also made to publications and documents of other intergovernmental bodies such as OECD, UNDP, UNESCO and UNCTAD, nongovernmental organizations and international scientific expert networks such as Réseau espérance de vie en santé (REVES). The Population Division of the Department for Economic and Social Information and Policy Analysis of the United Nations, hereinafter referred to as United Nations Population Division, was the main source for estimates relating to demographic indicators including life expectancy at birth and infant mortality. A number of statistical values such as the elderly support ratio were derived from

those estimates, but otherwise no attempt was made, for the present report, to refine figures taken from recognized international sources and research publications.

Diseases/conditions were assessed according to their effect on people's health at different stages of life, i.e. children, school-age children and adolescents, adults and the elderly. The available data were selected, reviewed, assembled and analysed and the findings synthesized to provide a reasonably accurate assessment. It was not possible to derive global estimates in respect of a number of crucial indicators, nor to arrive at regional estimates, although efforts will be made to do so in future issues of The World Health Report.

Because many of WHO's activities in different fields are interdependent, the programmes were clustered and their activities, products and other outputs synthesized according to objectives and target age groups. The aim being to provide a global overview of WHO's work during the year 1994, no account was taken of the organizational level at which activities were carried out, i.e. country, regional or interregional.

For analytical purposes WHO's 189 Member States were grouped according to the following classification used by the United Nations (as of August 1994). The designations used for groupings of countries in the text and tables are intended solely for statistical and analytical convenience and do not necessarily express a judgement about the stage reached by a particular country in the development process.

Developed market economies. North America, northern, southern and western Europe (excluding Bosnia and Herzegovina, Croatia, Cyprus, Malta,

Slovenia, The Former Yugoslav Republic of Macedonia, and Yugoslavia), Australia, Japan and New Zealand.

Developing countries. Latin America and the Caribbean, Africa, Asia and the Pacific (excluding Australia, Japan and New Zealand), Bosnia and Herzegovina, Croatia, Cyprus, Malta, Slovenia, The Former Yugoslav Republic of Macedonia, and Yugoslavia.

Least developed countries. Afghanistan, Bangladesh, Benin, Bhutan, Botswana, Burkina Faso, Burundi, Cambodia, Cape Verde, Central African Republic, Chad, Comoros, Djibouti, Equatorial Guinea, Ethiopia, Gambia, Guinea, Guinea-Bissau, Haiti, Kiribati, Lao People's Democratic Republic, Lesotho, Liberia, Madagascar, Malawi, Maldives, Mali, Mauritania, Mozambique, Myanmar, Nepal, Niger, Rwanda, Samoa, Sao Tome and Principe, Sierra Leone, Solomon Islands, Somalia, Sudan, Togo, Tuvalu, Uganda, United Republic of Tanzania, Vanuatu, Yemen, Zaire, Zambia.

Economies in transition. Albania, Bulgaria, Czech Republic, Hungary, Poland, Romania, Slovakia and former USSR (Baltic republics, Commonwealth of Independent States, Georgia).

Throughout the report "developed world" refers to countries classified as "developed market economies" and "economies in transition"; and "developing world" to "least developed countries" (LDCs) and "other developing countries".

A major constraint in the assessment of the global health situation relates to data on ***health status***. There are no clear *positive measures* of health. Since the early 1960s several attempts have been made to complement quantitative information on such factors as life expectancy by information concerning quality of life during the years lived, particularly given the increasing frequency of chronic nonlethal sensory, cognitive, osteoarticulatory and other impairments that accompany falling mortality. One major initiative is that of REVES (mentioned above), in developing techniques for calculating health expectancy adjusted for disability – e.g. disability-free life expectancy or DFLE. Another approach is that of the World Bank which, in close collaboration with WHO, has been devising a global burden of disease measure that combines loss of healthy life as a result of premature death with loss of healthy life due to disability, and is expressed in units of disability-adjusted life years or DALYs. However, since little information is at present available on disability and the data on incidence and prevalence of diseases are notoriously unreliable and enormously variable, this report is based on four distinct measures of ill-health only: mortality, incidence, prevalence and disability (long-term). Even data on negative measures such as mortality, morbidity and disability are not available for many countries, particularly in the developing world. Recourse was made to reasonably reliable data and estimates from a variety of administrative sources. For example, the United Nations Population Division biennially assesses the global situation and makes estimates of *numbers of deaths by age and sex* for many countries. Since the results of the 1994 assessment have not yet been published, results of the 1992 assessment were used for this report. Although mortality data are imperfect, they are nevertheless used to illustrate general patterns and orders of magnitude of major health problems. While caution is necessary in interpreting small differences in values of different groups, major differences may be considered indicative of actual disparities and trends.

In every country *cause-of-death* data

pose a problem. Underreporting, imprecise listing of causes and inaccurate diagnosis complicate both national and international studies of mortality. Furthermore attributing death to specific causes often results in overlap of underlying causes and also masks underlying conditions such as anaemia and nutritional deficiencies. In cases where data were lacking or inadequate, "guesstimates" were prepared in accordance with epidemiological and statistical principles and procedures, to ensure a reasonable degree of reliability.

Global values for mortality, morbidity and disability associated with a large number of diseases and conditions were determined following extensive consultation with experts within the Organization and at WHO collaborating centres concerning the quality and consistency of the estimates. Judicious use was made of available data from a variety of sources and the most recent data were reviewed, interpreted and extrapolated in a global context. As far as possible the disease categories were assigned codes according to the ninth revision of the International Classification of Diseases (ICD-9). Although coverage of diseases/conditions is fairly comprehensive in the report, it still falls far short of the total spectrum of causes covered by ICD. The resulting figures relating to 1993 indicate orders of magnitude of health problems but they lack the degree of precision necessary for disease-specific analysis.

Since 1990 WHO has been preparing global and regional estimates of mortality and morbidity by diseases/conditions, based on official country data supplemented by reliable national and international estimates. The extensive use, in this report, of data based on estimates and other indirect approaches should not give the mistaken impression that the necessary data are already being collected by all developing and developed countries; rather it is a matter of concern that use of such estimates may detract from the current efforts being made to compile accurate and timely data on health indicators in the devel-

oping world. Empirical data continue to be essential for identifying problems and working out solutions in the area of health development.

It would thus be appreciated if readers would send their comments and suggestions for improving the quality of the estimates used in this report and thereby assist WHO by suggesting more reliable data sources for use in the future.

Primary sources of data

Table A – Basic indicators gives data on key health and health-related indicators relating to the world health situation. It contains data for 1993 or for the latest available year during the period 1990-1992 in respect of the 189 WHO Member States (listed in *Annex 1*). Data for most of the indicators were assembled by WHO from the various sources listed; data concerning health status and health care were taken from WHO publications or are estimates made by WHO programmes on the basis of information supplied by Member States. Although every effort was made to standardize the data for international comparisons, they may not always be comparable between countries. Thus care must be taken in interpreting the values.

Table B – Analytical tabulations as well as *Tables 1-6* and *Figs 1-6* in the report are based on the values given in *Table A*. Figures refer to all 189 Member States, which in 1993 had an estimated population of 5.6 billion, or 99.7% of the world population. The population data are estimates of the United Nations Population Division following the 1992 population assessment. These figures serve as denominators for various rates and weights used for computing the aggregate values in *Table B*. Further details are given in the reference works listed in each case under *Source*.

Maps 1-6 relating respectively to poliomyelitis, tuberculosis, cholera, malaria, leprosy and HIV/AIDS are based on data compiled by WHO technical programmes.

1. Population and demography

Data for population size, growth rate, age and sex distribution, median age; population in urban areas and agglomerations >10 million; infant mortality rate, life expectancy at birth, total fertility rate; elderly support ratio (number of persons aged 65 or over per 100 persons aged 20-64).
Sources:
(a) *World population prospects, 1992 revision.* New York, United Nations, 1993. [Values for republics of former USSR were obtained from UNFPA.]
(b) *World population 1950-2025, 1992 revision.* New York, United Nations, 1993. [Database.]
(c) *The state of world population 1994.* New York, UNFPA, 1994.
(d) *World urbanization prospects, 1992 revision.* New York, United Nations, 1993.

2. Health status

2.1 *Mortality, morbidity and disability, selected causes.*
Source: WHO.

2.2 *Annual number of reported cases*
refers to the number of cases of tuberculosis, malaria, poliomyelitis, measles and neonatal tetanus (target diseases) occurring in 1993 and reported by WHO Member States by the end of 1994.
Source: WHO.

2.3 *Causes of deaths among children under age 5.*
Source: WHO.

2.4 *Under-5 mortality rate* refers to the annual number of deaths of children under 5 years per 1 000 live births. More specifically, it measures the probability of dying between birth and exactly 5 years of age.
Source: UNICEF. *The state of the world's children 1994.* New York, Oxford University Press, 1994.

2.5 *Age-specific death rates* for age groups 0-4, 20-49 (male), 20-49 (female), 65-74 and 75 years and above and *crude death rates* (*sources 1a* and *1b* – supplementary tabulations).
Source: WHO.

2.6 *Age and sex standardized death rate* is obtained by applying the age- and sex-specific death rates of a given population to a standard population. In this report the standard population used is the average world population for the years 1990-1995 (*source 1b*) estimated at 5.6 billion.
Source: WHO.

2.7 *Disability-free life expectancy* (DFLE) refers to the average number of years an individual is expected to live free of disability if current patterns of mortality and disability continue to apply.
Source: REVES. *Global assessment in positive health-contribution of the network on Health Expectancy and the Disability Process.* Montpellier, INSERM, 1994. (Unpublished document).

2.8 *Maternal mortality rate* is the number of maternal deaths attributed to complications of pregnancy and childbirth (within 42 days of termination of pregnancy) occurring over a year, per 100 000 live births in that year. In view of the paucity of the data and limitations in the estimation procedures, the data for 1993 on maternal mortality in *Table A* are presented in five broad categories: less than 25; 25-99; 100-249; 500 or more.
Source: WHO.

2.9 *Percentage of live births with low birth weight* refers to the number of newborns weighing less than 2.5 kg at birth in a given year per 100 live births in that year.
Source: WHO.

2.10 *Prevalence of malnutrition under age 5* refers to the percentage of children under 5 years who have a weight that is below minus two standard deviations from the median weight-for-age of the reference population.
Source: World Bank. *World development report 1994.* New York, Oxford University Press, 1994.

3. Health care and environment

3.1 *Physicians* are defined as graduates of a faculty or school of medicine in any medical field (practice, teaching, administration, research, laboratory, etc).
Sources:
(a) WHO.
(b) World Bank. *Social indicators of development 1994.* Baltimore, Johns Hopkins University Press, 1994. [For Japan and USA.]

3.2 *Nurses* are defined as all persons who have completed a programme of basic nursing education and are qualified and registered or authorized by the country to provide responsible and competent service for the promotion of health, prevention of illness, care of the sick and rehabilitation.
Source: WHO.

3.3 *Prenatal care* refers to the percentage of pregnant women who have had at least one consultation during pregnancy with a trained health worker. Since the number of pregnant women is generally not available, the number of live births is used as the denominator. In view of limitations in the estimation procedures, coverage data in *Table A* are presented in five broad categories: less than 40%; 40-59%; 60-79%; 80-89%; 90% or more.
Source: WHO.

3.4 *Deliveries attended* refers to the percentage of deliveries attended by personnel trained to give the necessary supervision, care and advice to women during pregnancy, labour and the postpartum period, to conduct deliveries on their own responsibility and to care for the newborn and the infant.
Source: WHO.

3.5 *Oral rehydration salts and/or recommended home fluid use rate* refers to the proportion of diarrhoea episodes in children under age 5 reported to have received oral rehydration salts (ORS) and/or a recommended home fluid (RHF).
Source: WHO.

3.6 *Immunization coverage for BCG, DPT3, OPV3 and measles* refers respectively to the percentages of infants surviving to age 1 who have been fully immunized with BCG, a third dose of diphtheria-pertussis-tetanus vaccine, a third dose of oral polio vaccine and with measles vaccine. *Immunization coverage for TT2* refers to the percentage of pregnant women immunized with two or more doses of tetanus toxoid given during pregnancy.
Source: WHO.

3.7 **Access to safe water** refers to the percentage of the population with safe drinking-water available in the home or with reasonable access to treated surface waters and untreated but uncontaminated water such as that from protected boreholes, springs and sanitary wells.
Access to adequate sanitation refers to the percentage population with at least adequate excreta-disposal facilities that can effectively prevent human, animal and insect contact with excreta.
Sources:
(a) WHO.
(b) UNICEF. *The state of the world's children 1994.* New York, Oxford University Press, 1994.

3.8 **Health expenditure per capita** refers to expenditure – public, parastatal (including social insurance) and private – incurred in preventive and curative health services for individuals and in public health programmes.
Source: *Global domestic expenditures on health.* Cambridge, Harvard School of Public Health, 1993 (Health Transition Working Paper Series No. 93.09).

3.9 **Central government expenditure for health** refers to public expenditure by government offices, departments, establishments and other bodies that are agencies or instruments of the central authority of a country on hospitals, maternity centres, dental centres and clinics with a major medical component; on national health and medical insurance schemes; and on family planning and preventive care. Where 1992 figures were not available, the most recent values are given.
Source: World Bank. *World development report 1994.* New York, Oxford University Press, 1994.

4. Education

4.1 **Adult literacy rate** refers to the percentage of persons aged 15 years and over who can, with understanding, both read and write a short simple statement on everyday life. For *Table B*, country data are weighted by the 1992 adult population for adult literacy and by the 1992 female adult population for female adult literacy.
Source: *World education report 1993.* Paris, Unesco, 1993.

4.2 **Gross primary enrolment ratio**. Figures for developing countries other than LDCs were estimated from data in source table.
Source: *World education report 1993.* Paris, Unesco, 1993.

4.3 **Percentage of drop-outs from primary education** refers to the number of pupils at primary level who do not reach grade 4, divided by the number of new entrants to grade 1. Figures for developing countries other than LDCs were estimated from data in source table.
Source: Unesco. *Statistical issues.* February 1992, Division of Statistics. (Document STE.8).

4.4 **Higher enrolment/primary enrolment ratio** refers to ratio of the number of students enrolled at the third level of education to the number enrolled at the primary level. Figures for developing countries other than LDCs were estimated from data in source table.
Source: *World education report 1993.* Paris, Unesco, 1993.

4.5 **Public education expenditure** and **percentage of gross national product** (GNP).
Source: *World education report 1993.* Paris, Unesco, 1993.

5. Economy

5.1 **Gross domestic product (GDP), average annual growth rate of GDP per capita, GNP, average annual growth rate of GNP.**
Sources:
(a) *World economic and social survey 1994.* New York, United Nations, 1994.
(b) World Bank. *World development report 1994.* New York, Oxford University Press, 1994.
(c) World Bank. *Social indicators of development 1994.* Baltimore, Johns Hopkins University Press, 1994.

5.2 **External debt/GDP ratio**
Source: *World economic outlook*, October 1994. Washington DC, IMF, 1994.

5.3 **Public expenditure on defence per capita**.
Source: Sivarld SL. *World military and social expenditure 1993.* Washington DC, United States Government Printing Office, 1994.

Table A1. Basic indicators

Estimates are obtained or derived from relevant WHO programmes or from responsible international agencies for the areas of their concern[a]

Member States	Age and sex standardized death rate (per 100 000) 1990-1995	Life expectancy at birth 1993	Infant mortality rate 1993	Under-5 mortality rate 1992	Total (000) 1993	% aged 65 years and above 1993	% in urban areas 1992	Total fertility rate 1990-1995	US $ 1992	Average annual growth (%) 1980-1992	Both sexes	Female	Health expenditure per capita US$ 1990
WHO Member States meeting all three health-for-all targets[b]													
Africa													
Mauritius	751	70	21	24	1 109	5.6	41	2	2 700	5.6	80	75	100
Americas													
Argentina	679	71	29	24	33 487	9.4	87	2.8	6 050	−0.9	95	95	137
Canada	466	78	7	8	27 755	11.9	78	1.8	20 710	1.8	...	...	1 945
Chile	656	72	17	18	13 813	6.2	85	2.7	2 730	3.7	93	93	100
Colombia	747	69	37	20	33 985	4.4	71	2.7	1 330	1.4	87	86	51
Costa Rica	479	76	14	16	3 270	4.5	48	3.1	1 960	0.8	93	93	132
Cuba	507	76	14	11	10 907	8.8	74	1.9	...	...	94	93	...
El Salvador	847	66	48	63	5 517	4	45	4	1 170	0	73	70	58
Jamaica	585	74	14	14	2 495	6.5	54	2.4	1 340	0.2	98	99	83
Mexico	698	70	35	33	89 998	3.9	74	3.2	3 470	−0.2	88	85	89
Panama	604	73	21	20	2 563	5	54	2.9	2 420	−1.2	89	88	142
Paraguay	831	67	47	34	4 643	3.6	49	4.3	1 380	−0.7	90	88	35
Trinidad and Tobago	682	71	20	22	1 279	5.6	65	2.7	3 940	−2.6	...	...	180
United States of America	520	76	8	10	257 840	12.7	76	2.1	23 240	1.7	...	...	2 765
Uruguay	652	72	20	22	3 149	12	89	2.3	3 340	−1	96	96	123
Venezuela	702	70	33	24	20 618	4	91	3.1	2 910	−0.8	88	90	88
Eastern Mediterranean													
Iran (Islamic Republic of)	832	67	42	58	63 180	3.7	58	6	2 200	−1.4	54	43	44
Jordan	821	68	36	30	4 440	2.7	69	5.7	...	...	80	70	55
Kuwait	521	75	12	17	1 825	1.4	93	3.7	...	...	73	67	541
Lebanon	808	69	34	44	2 901	5.4	86	3.1	...	...	80	73	...
Oman	750	70	30	31	1 697	2.8	12	6.7	6 480	4.1	...	...	209
Saudi Arabia	768	69	31	40	16 472	2.7	78	6.4	7 510	−3.3	62	48	260
Syrian Arab Republic	858	67	40	40	13 762	2.7	51	6.1	...	...	65	51	41
Tunisia	828	68	43	38	8 579	4.3	57	3.4	1 720	1.3	65	56	76
United Arab Emirates	667	71	22	22	1 709	2	82	4.5	22 020	−4.3	...	...	472
Europe													
Albania	583	73	24	34	3 338	5.5	36	2.7	...	...	...	...	26
Austria	527	76	8	9	7 805	15.4	59	1.5	22 380	2	...	...	1 711
Belgium	525	76	8	11	10 010	15.4	96	1.7	20 880	2	...	...	1 449
Bulgaria	692	72	13	20	8 926	13.9	69	1.8	1 330	1.2	...	...	121
Denmark	538	76	7	8	5 169	15.6	85	1.7	26 000	2.1	...	...	1 588
Estonia	723	72	13	24	1 578	12.2	72	2	2 760[c]	−2.3[c]	100	100	228
Finland	544	76	6	7	5 020	13.8	60	1.8	21 970	2	...	...	2 046
France	491	77	7	9	57 379	14.5	73	1.8	22 260	1.7	...	...	1 869
Germany	530	76	7	8	80 606	14.7	86	1.5	23 030	...	...	...	1 511
Greece	458	77	9	9	10 208	14.7	63	1.5	7 290	1	93	89	359
Hungary	788	71	14	16	10 493	13.6	66	1.8	2 970	0.2	...	...	185
Ireland	545	75	7	6	3 481	11.5	58	2.1	12 210	3.4	...	...	876
Israel	505	77	9	11	5 411	9.5	92	2.9	13 220	1.9	...	...	480
Italy	478	77	8	10	57 866	15	70	1.3	20 460	2.2	97	96	1 426
Latvia	730	72	10	26	2 669	12.6	72	2	1 930[c]	0.2[c]	100	99	220
Lithuania	646	73	10	20	3 760	11.6	70	2	1 310[c]	−1.0[c]	98	98	159
Netherlands	470	78	7	7	15 270	12.9	89	1.7	20 480	1.7	...	...	1 501
Norway	481	77	8	8	4 310	16.2	76	2	25 820	2.2	...	...	1 835
Poland	707	72	15	16	38 518	10.5	63	2.1	1 910	0.1	...	...	84
Portugal	562	75	12	13	9 870	13.8	35	1.5	7 450	3.1	85	82	383
Romania	764	70	23	28	23 377	11	55	2.1	1 130	−1.1	97	95	58
Spain	463	78	7	9	39 153	14.2	79	1.4	13 970	2.9	...	...	831
Sweden	452	78	6	7	8 692	17.6	84	2.1	27 010	1.5	...	...	2 343
Switzerland	450	78	7	9	6 862	15.1	62	1.7	36 080	1.4	...	...	2 520
United Kingdom	516	76	8	9	57 826	15.6	89	1.9	17 790	2.4	...	...	1 039
South-East Asia													
Democratic People's Republic of Korea	706	71	25	33	23 054	4.4	60	2.4	...	...	...	...	...
Sri Lanka	659	72	24	19	17 894	5.6	22	2.5	540	2.6	88	84	18
Thailand	753	69	27	33	56 868	4.2	23	2.2	1 840	6	93	90	72

Member States	Age and sex standardized death rate (per 100 000) 1990-1995	Life expectancy at birth 1993	Infant mortality rate 1993	Under-5 mortality rate 1992	Total (000) 1993	Population		Total fertility rate 1990-1995	GNP per capita		Adult literacy rate 1990		Health expenditure per capita US$ 1990
						% aged 65 years and above 1993	% in urban areas 1992		US $ 1992	Average annual growth (%) 1980-1992	Both sexes	Female	
Western Pacific													
Australia	478	77	8	9	17 843	11.5	85	1.9	17 260	1.6	...	...	1 294
China	699	71	27	43	1 205 181	6	28	2.2	470	7.6	78	68	11
Japan	420	79	5	6	124 959	13	77	1.7	28 190	3.6	...	...	1 538
Malaysia	694	71	14	19	19 239	3.8	45	3.6	2 790	3.2	78	70	71
New Zealand	526	76	9	10	3 487	11	84	2.1	12 300	0.6	...	...	925
Philippines	943	65	39	60	66 543	3.2	44	3.9	770	−1	90	90	15
Republic of Korea	747	71	21	9	44 508	5.1	74	1.8	6 790	8.5	96	94	365
Singapore	568	75	7	7	2 798	6.1	100	1.7	15 730	5.3	...	...	215
Viet Nam	977	65	38	49	70 902	4.8	20	3.9	...	...	88	84	3
WHO Member States not meeting all three health-for-all targets[b]													
Africa													
Angola	1 971	47	123	292	10 276	2.9	30	7.2	...	...	42	29	...
Benin	1 841	46	85	147	5 075	2.9	40	7.1	410	−0.7	23	16	19
Burkina Faso	1 827	48	116	150	9 788	3	17	6.5	300	1	18	9	7
Burundi	1 833	48	105	179	5 995	3	6	6.8	210	1.3	50	40	30
Cameroon	1 366	56	64	117	12 547	3.6	42	5.7	820	−1.5	54	43	27
Central African Republic	1 906	47	104	179	3 258	3.9	48	6.2	410	−1.5	38	25	18
Chad	1 883	48	121	209	6 010	3.6	34	5.9	220	3.4	30	18	12
Congo	1 603	51	81	110	2 441	3.4	42	6.3	1 030	−0.8	57	44	50
Côte d'Ivoire	1 612	51	91	124	13 397	2.6	42	7.4	670	−4.7	54	40	28
Gabon	1 571	54	93	158	1 279	5.8	47	5.3	4 450	−3.7	61	49	164
Ghana	1 363	56	80	170	16 446	2.9	35	6	450	−0.1	60	51	15
Guinea	2 101	45	133	230	6 306	2.6	27	7	510	...	24	13	17
Guinea-Bissau	2 182	44	139	239	1 028	4.2	21	5.8	220	1.6	37	24	16
Kenya	1 176	59	65	74	26 090	2.9	25	6.3	310	0.2	69	59	16
Liberia	1 371	55	126	217	2 845	3.7	47	6.8	...	...	40	29	14
Madagascar	1 452	56	110	168	13 259	2.9	25	6.6	230	−2.4	80	73	7
Malawi	2 040	45	140	226	10 694	2.6	12	7.6	210	−0.1	...	...	11
Mali	1 985	46	158	220	10 137	2.6	25	7.1	310	−2.7	32	24	15
Mauritania	1 851	48	116	206	2 206	3.1	49	6.5	530	−0.8	36	27	18
Mozambique	1 928	47	143	287	15 322	3.3	30	6.5	60	−3.6	33	21	5
Namibia	1 241	59	69	79	1 584	3.5	29	6	1 610	−1	...	...	45
Niger	1 954	47	123	320	8 529	2.5	21	7.1	280	−4.3	28	17	16
Nigeria	1 559	53	95	191	119 328	2.6	37	6.4	320	−0.4	51	40	10
Rwanda	1 955	47	109	222	7 789	2.3	6	8.5	250	−0.6	50	37	10
Senegal	1 751	49	79	145	7 948	2.9	41	6.1	780	0.1	38	25	29
Sierra Leone	2 216	43	142	249	4 494	3.1	34	6.5	160	−1.4	21	11	4
Togo	1 427	55	85	137	3 885	3.2	29	6.6	390	−1.8	43	31	18
Uganda	2 310	43	101	185	19 246	2.5	12	7.3	170	...	48	35	8
United Republic of Tanzania	1 653	51	100	176	28 783	2.5	22	6.8	110[d]	0.0[d]	...	...	4
Zaire	1 603	51	93	188	41 166	2.9	28	6.7	...	−1.8	72	61	5
Zambia	2 131	45	82	202	8 885	2.3	42	6.3	...	...	73	65	17
Zimbabwe	1 348	56	61	86	10 898	2.8	30	5.3	570	−0.9	67	60	39
Americas													
Haiti	1 373	57	86	133	6 893	4	30	4.8	...	−2.4	53	47	27
Eastern Mediterranean													
Afghanistan	2 294	44	161	257	20 547	2.7	19	6.9	...	...	29	14	...
Pakistan	1 215	59	98	137	128 057	2.9	33	6.2	420	3.1	35	21	12
Somalia	1 927	47	121	211	9 517	2.7	25	7	...	...	24	14	8
Sudan	1 600	52	98	166	27 407	2.9	23	6	...	...	27	12	34
Yemen	1 579	53	105	177	12 977	2.4	31	7.2	...	...	...[e]	...[f]	20
South-East Asia													
Bangladesh	1 554	53	107	127	122 210	3	18	4.7	220	1.8	35	22	7
Bhutan	1 851	49	125	201	1 650	3.3	6	5.9	180	6.3	38	25	10
Myanmar	1 312	58	81	113	44 613	4	25	4.2	...	...	81	72	...
Nepal	1 534	54	98	128	21 086	3.1	12	5.5	170	2	26	13	7

Member States	Age and sex standardized death rate (per 100 000) 1990-1995	Life expectancy at birth 1993	Infant mortality rate 1993	Under-5 mortality rate 1992	Population Total (000) 1993	Population % aged 65 years and above 1993	Population % in urban areas 1992	Total fertility rate 1990-1995	GNP per capita US $ 1992	GNP per capita Average annual growth (%) 1980-1992	Adult literacy rate 1990 Both sexes	Adult literacy rate 1990 Female	Health expenditure per capita US$ 1990
Western Pacific													
Cambodia	1 692	51	115	184	8 997	2.7	12	4.5	...	...	35	22	...
Lao People's Democratic Republic	1 712	51	96	145	4 605	3	20	6.7	250	...	...	...	5
Papua New Guinea	1 670	56	53	77	4 149	2.6	17	4.9	950	0	52	38	37

WHO Member States meeting at least one of the values above the health-for-all targets[b]

Member States	Age and sex standardized death rate (per 100 000) 1990-1995	Life expectancy at birth 1993	Infant mortality rate 1993	Under-5 mortality rate 1992	Population Total (000) 1993	Population % aged 65 years and above 1993	Population % in urban areas 1992	Total fertility rate 1990-1995	GNP per capita US $ 1992	GNP per capita Average annual growth (%) 1980-1992	Adult literacy rate 1990 Both sexes	Adult literacy rate 1990 Female	Health expenditure per capita US$ 1990
Africa													
Algeria	913	66	60	72	27 070	3.5	53	4.9	1 840	−0.5	57	46	149
Botswana	1 127	61	60	58	1 352	3.3	27	5.1	2 790	6.1	74	65	139
Cape Verde	858	68	42	...	395	4.1	...	4.3	850	3	67	...	64
Lesotho	1 132	61	78	156	1 882	3.9	21	4.7	590	−0.5	...	...	26
South Africa	1 028	63	52	70	40 774	4	50	4.1	2 670	0.1	...	...	141
Americas													
Bahamas	652	72	22	...	268	4.1	...	2	12 070	1	...	...	...
Barbados	519	76	10	...	260	11.9	...	1.8	6 540	1	...	...	323
Bolivia	1 102	61	84	118	7 705	3.8	52	4.6	680	−1.5	78	71	25
Brazil	847	66	56	65	156 578	5	76	2.7	2 770	0.4	81	80	146
Dominican Republic	805	68	56	50	7 621	3.7	62	3.3	1 050	−0.5	83	82	38
Ecuador	836	67	57	59	11 310	3.9	58	3.6	1 070	−0.3	87	84	44
Guatemala	916	65	49	76	10 029	3.4	40	5.4	980	−1.5	55	47	27
Guyana	923	65	48	...	816	3.9	...	2.5	330	−5.6	96	95	42
Honduras	871	66	59	58	5 628	3.3	45	4.9	580	−0.3	73	71	52
Nicaragua	831	66	57	76	4 114	3.1	61	5	340	−5.3	...	...	34
Peru	944	64	76	65	22 913	4	71	3.6	950	−2.8	85	79	61
Suriname	732	70	28	...	446	4.3	...	2.7	4 280	−3.6	95	95	93
Eastern Mediterranean													
Bahrain	608	71	14	...	548	2.4	...	3.8	...	−3.8	77	69	324
Cyprus	476	77	9	...	723	10.2	...	2.3	9 820	5	...	...	64
Egypt	1 085	62	55	55	56 060	4.1	44	4.1	640	1.8	48	34	28
Iraq	879	67	54	80	19 918	2.9	73	5.7	...	...	60	49	...
Libyan Arab Jamahiriya	1 021	63	68	104	5 048	2.5	84	6.4	...	...	64	50	...
Morocco	1 010	63	68	61	26 954	3.8	47	4.4	1 030	1.4	50	38	26
Qatar	628	70	26	...	466	1.5	...	4.4	16 750	−11.2	...	...	630
Europe													
Armenia	...	...	...	34	...	...	...	2.6[g]	780[c]	...	99	98	152
Azerbaijan	...	...	...	53	...	...	...	2.8[g]	740[c]	...	97	96	99
Belarus	...	...	...	23	...	...	...	2[g]	2 930[c]	...	98	97	157
Czech Republic	...	...	...	12	...	...	...	...	2 450	...	...	...	...
Georgia	...	...	...	29	...	...	...	2.3[g]	850[c]	...	99	99	152
Iceland	442	78	5	...	263	10.6	...	2.2	23 880	1.5	...	...	1 884
Kazakhstan	...	...	...	50	...	...	...	3[g]	1 680[c]	...	98	96	154
Kyrgyzstan	...	...	...	60	...	...	...	4[g]	820[c]	...	97	96	118
Luxembourg	538	75	8	...	380	13.9	...	1.6	35 160	3.3	...	...	1 662
Malta	511	76	9	...	361	10.8	...	2.1	...	3.8	...	...	349
Republic of Moldova	...	...	...	36	...	...	...	2.6[g]	1 300[c]	...	96	94	143
Russian Federation	...	...	...	32	...	...	...	2.1[g]	2 510[c]	...	99	98	159
Slovakia	...	...	...	14	...	...	...	...	1 930	...	...	...	...
Turkey	841	67	57	87	59 577	4.6	64	3.5	1 980	2.9	81	71	76
Ukraine	...	...	...	25	...	...	...	2[g]	1 820[c]	...	98	97	131
Uzbekistan	...	...	...	68	...	...	...	...	690[c]	...	97	96	116
South-East Asia													
India	1 145	61	86	124	896 567	4.7	26	3.9	310	3.1	48	34	21
Indonesia	1 009	63	65	111	194 617	4.2	30	3.1	670	4	82	75	12
Maldives	997	64	54	78	234	4.3	...	6.2	500	6.8	...	...	...
Mongolia	996	64	59	80	2 371	3.2	59	4.6	...	...	...	...	58

Member States	Age and sex standardized death rate (per 100 000) 1990-1995	Life expectancy at birth 1993	Infant mortality rate 1993	Under-5 mortality rate 1992	Population Total (000) 1993	Population % aged 65 years and above 1993	Population % in urban areas 1992	Total fertility rate 1990-1995	GNP per capita US $ 1992	GNP per capita Average annual growth (%) 1980-1992	Adult literacy rate 1990 Both sexes	Adult literacy rate 1990 Female	Health expenditure per capita US$ 1990
Western Pacific													
Brunei Darussalam	510	74	8	...	276	4.7	...	3.1	...	...	...	...	...
Fiji	681	72	23	...	747	3.7	...	3	2 010	0.3	...	...	70
Solomon Islands	790	70	27	...	354	2.8	...	5.4	710	3.3	...	...	117

WHO Member States for which insufficient data are available for life expectancy, infant mortality and under-5 mortality

Member States	Age and sex standardized death rate (per 100 000) 1990-1995	Life expectancy at birth 1993	Infant mortality rate 1993	Under-5 mortality rate 1992	Population Total (000) 1993	Population % aged 65 years and above 1993	Population % in urban areas 1992	Total fertility rate 1990-1995	GNP per capita US $ 1992	GNP per capita Average annual growth (%) 1980-1992	Adult literacy rate 1990 Both sexes	Adult literacy rate 1990 Female	Health expenditure per capita US$ 1990
Africa													
Comoros	1 397	56	88	...	607	2.3	...	7.1	510	−1.3	...	...	28
Equatorial Guinea	1 827	48	116	...	379	4	...	5.9	330	...	50	37	28
Eritrea	...	...	...	208	...	...	...	...	...	...	...	...	...
Ethiopia	...	...	...	208	...	...	13	...	110	−1.9	...	...	...
Gambia	2 057	45	131	...	932	2.9	...	6.1	370	−0.4	27	16	22
Sao Tome and Principe	...	...	...	...	127	...	...	...	360	−3	...	...	38
Seychelles	...	...	...	...	72	...	...	...	5 460	3.2	...	...	289
Swaziland	1 265	58	72	...	814	3.3	...	4.9	1 090	1.6	...	...	64
Americas													
Antigua and Barbuda	...	...	...	...	67	...	...	...	5 980	5	...	...	241
Belize	...	...	...	...	202	...	...	...	2 220	2.6	...	...	120
Dominica	...	...	...	...	72	...	...	...	2 520	4.6	...	...	192
Grenada	...	...	...	...	92	...	...	...	2 310	...	...	...	133
Saint Kitts and Nevis	...	...	...	...	42	...	...	...	3 990	5.7	...	...	212
Saint Lucia	...	...	...	...	139	...	...	...	2 920	...	...	...	169
Saint Vincent and the Grenadines	...	...	...	...	110	...	...	...	1 990	5	...	...	102
Eastern Mediterranean													
Djibouti	1 812	49	111	...	481	2.7	...	6.6	...	...	...	...	...
Europe													
Bosnia and Herzegovina	...	...	...	...	...	...	...	...	...	...	...	...	...
Croatia	...	...	...	...	...	...	...	...	...	...	...	...	...
Monaco	...	...	...	...	28	...	...	...	...	...	...	...	...
San Marino	...	...	...	...	23	...	...	...	...	...	...	...	...
Slovenia	...	...	...	...	...	...	...	...	6 540	...	...	...	...
Tajikistan	...	...	...	85	...	...	...	5.4 g	490 c	...	98	97	100
The Former Yugoslav Republic of Macedonia	...	...	...	...	...	...	...	...	...	...	...	...	...
Turkmenistan	...	...	...	91	...	...	...	4.6 g	1 230 c	...	98	97	125
Yugoslavia	...	...	...	...	...	...	...	...	...	...	...	...	...
Western Pacific													
Cook Islands	...	...	...	...	17	...	...	...	...	...	...	...	...
Kiribati	...	...	...	...	75	...	...	...	700	...	...	...	...
Marshall Islands	...	...	...	...	51	...	...	...	...	...	...	...	...
Micronesia (Federated States of)	...	...	...	...	114	...	...	...	...	...	...	...	...
Nauru	...	...	...	...	10	...	...	...	...	...	...	...	...
Niue	...	...	...	...	2	...	...	...	...	...	...	...	...
Samoa	...	...	...	...	158	...	...	...	940	...	...	...	20
Tonga	...	...	...	...	98	...	...	...	1 480	...	...	...	63
Tuvalu	...	...	...	...	13	...	...	...	...	...	...	...	...
Vanuatu	...	...	...	...	161	...	...	...	1 210	...	...	...	67

a Figures in italics are the latest available and not for the year(s) specified.
b The three targets in WHO's strategy for health for all by the year 2000 relating to health status are: life expectancy at birth above 60 years; infant mortality rate below 50 per 1 000 live births; under-5 mortality rate below 70 per 1 000 live births. Estimates of under-5 mortality rate for less populous countries have been excluded.
c Estimates for republics of former USSR are subject to more than the usual range of uncertainty and should be regarded as preliminary.
d GNP data are for United Republic of Tanzania (mainland) only.
e Previous figures for adult literacy (both sexes) were: former Democratic Yemen (39.1); former Yemen Arab Republic (38.5).
f Previous figures for adult literacy (female) were: former Democratic Yemen (26.1); former Yemen Arab Republic (26.3).
g Estimates for republics of former USSR were obtained from UNFPA.
... Data not available or not applicable.

Table A2. Basic indicators

Estimates are obtained or derived from relevant WHO programmes or from responsible international agencies for the areas of their concern[a]

Member States	% of total central government expenditure for health 1991-1992	Prenatal care (% of live births) 1990	Deliveries attended (% of live births) 1990	Maternal mortality (per 100 000 live births) 1993	% of live births with low birth weight 1990	Immunization coverage (%) 1993[b]					ORS and/or RHF use rate[c] (%) 1993
						Children immunized by age 12 months				Pregnant women	
						BCG	DPT3	OPV 3	Measles[d]	Tetanus toxoid	
WHO Member States meeting all three health-for-all targets[e]											
Africa											
Mauritius	8.1	≥90	85	25-99	9	87	88	88	84	79	...
Americas											
Argentina	3	40-59	92	25-99	8	96	79	80	95	...	80
Canada	5.2	≥90	100	<25	6	...	85	85	85	...	...
Chile	11.1	≥90	98	25-99	7	97	94	94	93	...	90
Colombia	...	60-79	71	25-99	10	94	83	85	94	14	40
Costa Rica	32	≥90	97	25-99	7	97	86	87	82	90	78
Cuba	...	≥90	99	25-99	8	97	100	97	96	55	80
El Salvador	7.3	60-79	85	250-499	11	79	79	79	86	47	45
Jamaica	...	≥90	90	25-99	11	99	91	93	80	...	10
Mexico	1.9	60-79	69	25-99	12	95	91	92	91	42	87
Panama	21.8	60-79	84	25-99	10	91	81	83	92	24	70
Paraguay	4.3	80-89	66	100-249	8	95	79	80	96	87	52
Trinidad and Tobago	...	≥90	98	25-99	10	...	81	78	87	19	75
United States of America	16	≥90	99	<25	7	...	83	72	83	...	...
Uruguay	5	80-89	96	25-99	8	99	88	88	80	13	96
Venezuela	...	60-79	97	25-99	9	82	69	75	63	...	80
Eastern Mediterranean											
Iran (Islamic Republic of)	7.6	40-59	70	100-249	9	100	99	99	96	82	85
Jordan	5.2	80-89	87	25-99	7	...	94	94	88	31	53
Kuwait	...	≥90	97	<25	7	99	99	99	87	38	10
Lebanon	...	80-89	...	25-99	10	...	87	87	65	...	45
Oman	5.7	80-89	75	100-249	10	99	96	96	94	85	72
Saudi Arabia	...	80-89	90	25-99	7	94	94	94	92	62	90
Syrian Arab Republic	1.9	60-79	61	25-99	11	91	90	90	86	50	95
Tunisia	6.6	60-79	70	25-99	8	81	98	98	89	50	22
United Arab Emirates	...	≥90	99	25-99	6	98	90	90	90	...	81
Europe											
Albania	...	≥90	...	25-99	7	82	96	98	76	...	...
Austria	13	≥90	...	<25	6	...	90	90	60	...	...
Belgium	...	≥90	100	<25	6	...	85	100	67	...	...
Bulgaria	4.8	≥90	...	25-99	6	98	98	97	87	...	...
Denmark	1.1	≥90	100	<25	6	...	88	95	81	...	...
Estonia	...	...	...	25-99	...	99	79	84	74	...	...
Finland	3.2	≥90	100	<25	4	99	99	100	99	...	...
France	16	≥90	...	<25	5	78	89	92	76	...	...
Germany	...	≥90	100	<25	6	...	75	90	70	...	...
Greece	8.7	≥90	...	<25	6	...	54	77	76	...	...
Hungary	7.9	≥90	...	<25	9	100	99	99	99	...	...
Ireland	13	≥90	...	<25	4	...	65[f]	63	78	...	...
Israel	4.4	≥90	99	<25	7	...	91	91	96	...	...
Italy	...	≥90	100	<25	5	...	95[f]	98	50	...	...
Latvia	...	...	...	25-99	...	91	79	83	80	...	...
Lithuania	...	...	...	25-99	...	98	92	97	94	...	...
Netherlands	13.9	≥90	100	<25	4	...	97	97	95	...	...
Norway	10.3	≥90	100	<25	4	...	98	98	96	...	...
Poland	...	≥90	...	<25	8	95	95	95	95	...	...
Portugal	8	≥90	98	25-99	5	92	92	91	94	...	...
Romania	9.2	≥90	...	25-99	7	93	91	91	99	...	...
Spain	7	≥90	...	<25	4	...	87	88	90	...	...
Sweden	0.8	≥90	100	<25	5	...	99[f]	99	95	...	...
Switzerland	...	≥90	99	<25	5	...	89	95	83	...	...
United Kingdom	13.8	≥90	100	<25	7	...	91	93	92	...	...

Member States	% of total central government expenditure for health 1991-1992	Prenatal care (% of live births) 1990	Deliveries attended (% of live births) 1990	Maternal mortality (per 100 000 live births) 1993	% of live births with low birth weight 1990	Immunization coverage (%) 1993[b]					ORS and/or RHF use rate[c] (%) 1993
						Children immunized by age 12 months				Pregnant women	
						BCG	DPT3	OPV 3	Measles[d]	Tetanus toxoid	
South-East Asia											
Democratic People's Republic of Korea	...	≥90	99	25-99	...	99	90	99	99	97	85
Sri Lanka	4.8	60-79	94	25-99	25	88	90	89	86	84	76
Thailand	8.1	60-79	66	100-249	13	96	88	88	78	75	65
Western Pacific											
Australia	12.7	≥90	99	<25	6	...	95	72	86	...	...
China	...	80-89	95	100-249	9	93	95	95	94	2	22
Japan	...	≥90	100	<25	6	93	87	94[g]	69	...	...
Malaysia	5.9	60-79	98	25-99	10	100	87	89	84	86	*47*
New Zealand	12.1	≥90	100	<25	6	20	81	68	82	...	...
Philippines	4.1	60-79	55	100-249	15	90	88	89	88	70	59
Republic of Korea	1.2	80-89	89	25-99	9	72	74	74	93	...	...
Singapore	6.2	≥90	99	<25	7	98	92	92	87	...	...
Viet Nam	...	≥90	90	100-249	17	94	91	91	93	71	52
WHO Member States not meeting all three health-for-all targets[e]											
Africa											
Angola	...	<40	15	≥500	19	53	30	28	47	14	*48*
Benin	...	60-79	45	250-499	15	85	73	73	66	77	28
Burkina Faso	...	<40	41	≥500	21	63	76	76	41	34	15
Burundi	...	60-79	19	≥500	...	72	69	69	67	56	49
Cameroon	*3.4*	60-79	64	250-499	13	41	33	33	33	7	84
Central African Republic	...	60-79	66	≥500	15	85	45	45	32	81	*24*
Chad	...	<40	15	≥500	...	34	10	13	25	6	*15*
Congo	...	<40	...	250-499	16	63	54	54	47	53	*67*
Côte d'Ivoire	...	40-59	40	250-499	14	53	50	50	52	51	*16*
Gabon	...	60-79	79	250-499	12	97	66	66	65	52	*25*
Ghana	...	80-89	40	250-499	14	70	49	48	50	14	44
Guinea	...	<40	25	≥500	21	76	55	55	57	61	82
Guinea-Bissau	*1.4*	<40	...	≥500	20	100	65	64	52	41	26
Kenya	5.4	60-79	50	250-499	16	93	86	85	81	71	*69*
Liberia	...	80-89	58	250-499	...	...	...	...	...	...	15
Madagascar	6.6	60-79	58	≥500	10	82	65	63	50	36	26
Malawi	7.8	60-79	50	≥500	20	98	86	84	82	66	50
Mali	...	<40	30	≥500	17	77	46	46	51	45	41
Mauritania	...	<40	20	≥500	11	84	44	44	49	36	*54*
Mozambique	...	40-59	25	≥500	20	66	49	49	62	24	60
Namibia	9.7	80-89	68	250-499	12	91	69	83	76	45	75
Niger	...	<40	15	≥500	...	30	18	18	18	43	17
Nigeria	...	60-79	37	250-499	16	40	29	29	34	33	80
Rwanda	...	80-89	22	≥500	17	94	85	85	81	88	36
Senegal	...	60-79	41	≥500	11	69	52	52	46	30	27
Sierra Leone	9.6	<40	25	≥500	17	79	63	63	67	81	*60*
Togo	...	60-79	42	250-499	20	75	53	53	47	77	33
Uganda	...	80-89	38	≥500	...	98	71	70	68	83	45
United Republic of Tanzania	...	≥90	53	≥500	14	90	77	78	77	72	*83*
Zaire	...	...	...	≥500	15	65	32	31	31	29	46
Zambia	...	≥90	51	≥500	13	69	48	47	47	17	90
Zimbabwe	*7.6*	≥90	70	250-499	14	82	73	72	72	50	82
Americas											
Haiti	...	60-79	78	≥500	15	48	30	30	24	23	*20*
Eastern Mediterranean											
Afghanistan	...	<40	9	≥500	20	21	23	23	19	2	*26*
Pakistan	1	<40	35	250-499	25	87	74	74	71	46	59
Somalia	...	40-59	2	≥500	16	31	18	18	30	5	*78*
Sudan	...	60-79	69	≥500	15	61	51	51	49	9	47
Yemen	...	<40	16	≥500	19	57	54	54	51	12	*6*

Member States	% of total central government expenditure for health 1991-1992	Prenatal care (% of live births) 1990	Deliveries attended (% of live births) 1990	Maternal mortality (per 100 000 live births) 1993	% of live births with low birth weight 1990	Immunization coverage (%) 1993[b]					ORS and/or RHF use rate[c] (%) 1993
						Children immunized by age 12 months				Pregnant women	
						BCG	DPT3	OPV 3	Measles[d]	Tetanus toxoid	
South-East Asia											
Bangladesh	*4.8*	<40	7	≥500	50	95	74	92	71	73	26
Bhutan	4.8	<40	20	≥500	...	79	72	73	58	45	85
Myanmar	6.8	80-89	70	250-499	16	96	64	41	44	66	37
Nepal	4.7	<40	6	≥500	...	59	60	60	55	12	14
Western Pacific											
Cambodia	...	<40	...	≥500	...	57	35	36	37	22	*6*
Lao People's Democratic Republic	...	<40	20	≥500	18	42	25	26	46	24	55
Papua New Guinea	7.9	60-79	43	≥500	23	65	37	36	51	27	51
WHO Member States meeting at least one of the values above the health-for-all targets[e]											
Africa											
Algeria	...	<40	78	100-249	9	87	73	73	69	38	*27*
Botswana	4.7	≥90	77	100-249	8	50	59	58	58	46	64
Cape Verde	...	≥90	50	100-249	...	100	100	100	95	98	*5*
Lesotho	11.5	80-89	60	250-499	11	97	80	82	85	...	42
South Africa	...	≥90	90	25-99	12	66	79	79	85	26	...
Americas											
Bahamas	...	...	...	25-99	7	87	91	91	88	68	*54*
Barbados	...	≥90	98	25-99	10	95	86	88	52	100	*15*
Bolivia	8.2	40-59	55	250-499	12	84	81	83	81	47	*63*
Brazil	6.9	60-79	73	100-249	11	90	69	92	78	62	*63*
Dominican Republic	14	≥90	92	100-249	15	84	57	82	100	87	37
Ecuador	11	60-79	84	100-249	13	99	76	79	73	19	89
Guatemala	*9.9*	40-59	89	250-499	14	69	76	77	68	33	24
Guyana	...	<40	...	250-499	17	94	93	92	90	47	*31*
Honduras	...	60-79	81	250-499	9	92	94	95	94	48	70
Nicaragua	...	≥90	73	100-249	13	94	78	94	83	49	40
Peru	*5.6*	60-79	60	100-249	11	87	84	86	75	21	*31*
Suriname	...	≥90	91	100-249	13	...	76	73	61	99	63
Eastern Mediterranean											
Bahrain	...	≥90	97	25-99	6	...	96	96	90	48	73
Cyprus	...	≥90	98	...	6	...	95	95	83	57	60
Egypt	*2.8*	40-59	35	100-249	10	95	89	89	89	78	34
Iraq	...	40-59	60	25-99	15	99	84	84	83	55	*70*
Libyan Arab Jamahiriya	...	60-79	76	25-99	...	99	91	91	89	45	*80*
Morocco	3	<40	31	100-249	9	91	86	86	83	87	14
Qatar	...	≥90	99	25-99	5	99	90	90	87	...	*20*
Europe											
Armenia	...	...	...	25-99	...	88	85	92	93	...	...
Azerbaijan	...	...	...	<25	...	94	72	70	84	...	...
Belarus	...	...	...	25-99	...	94	86	91	96	...	...
Czech Republic	...	...	...	...	...	98	99	99	98	...	...
Georgia	...	...	...	25-99	...	63	45	45	58	...	...
Iceland	...	≥90	100	<25	3	...	98	99	98	...	...
Kazakhstan	...	...	...	25-99	...	93	76	69	91	...	...
Kyrgyzstan	...	...	...	25-99	...	95	60	69	93	...	...
Luxembourg	...	≥90	100	<25	4	...	90	90	80	...	...
Malta	...	...	...	<25	4	77	63	83	90	...	...
Republic of Moldova	...	...	...	25-99	...	96	87	97	92	...	...
Russian Federation	...	...	...	25-99	...	87	65	82	88	...	...
Slovakia	...	...	...	...	...	91	99	99	96	...	...
Turkey	3.5	40-59	76	25-99	8	59	65	65	62	20	...
Ukraine	...	...	...	...	...	89	90	91	94	...	...
Uzbekistan	...	...	...	25-99	...	89	58	51	91	...	...

Member States	% of total central government expenditure for health 1991-1992	Prenatal care (% of live births) 1990	Deliveries attended (% of live births) 1990	Maternal mortality (per 100 000 live births) 1993	% of live births with low birth weight 1990	Immunization coverage (%) 1993[b]					ORS and/or RHF use rate[c] (%) 1993
						Children immunized by age 12 months				Pregnant women	
						BCG	DPT3	OPV 3	Measles[d]	Tetanus toxoid	
South-East Asia											
India	1.6	40-59	32	250-499	33	92	90	90	85	78	*37*
Indonesia	2.8	60-79	40	250-499	14	94	89	95	93	67	78
Maldives	...	...	...	250-499	...	89	90	97	86	94	27
Mongolia	...	≥90	99	100-249	10	84	80	66	84	...	65
Western Pacific											
Brunei Darussalam	...	...	...	25-99	12	97	96	100	92	50	...
Fiji	...	≥90	96	25-99	12	100	99	100	93	6	100
Solomon Islands	...	...	...	250-499	20	83	76	74	76	65	60
WHO Member States for which insufficient data are available for life expectancy, infant mortality and under-5 mortality											
Africa											
Comoros	...	60-79	24	250-499	8	94	60	60	60	59	*70*
Equatorial Guinea	...	<40	58	≥500	...	75	76	76	70	57	*40*
Eritrea	...	...	...	...	...	...	...	...	...	...	...
Ethiopia	...	40-59	10	≥500	16	46	28	28	22	13	68
Gambia	...	≥90	...	≥500	20	97	81	84	66	69	51
Sao Tome and Principe	...	...	...	...	7	97	78	78	69	48	*50*
Seychelles	...	...	...	...	10	100	96	96	92	100	...
Swaziland	...	80-89	55	250-499	10	97	89	86	85	81	*85*
Americas											
Antigua and Barbuda	...	...	...	...	8	...	100	100	100	...	*50*
Belize	...	...	...	...	...	94	88	89	83	...	92
Dominica	...	...	...	...	10	99	99	99	99	...	*50*
Grenada	...	...	...	...	...	66	89	91	99	...	*70*
Saint Kitts and Nevis	...	...	...	...	10	...	100	100	100	...	*5*
Saint Lucia	...	...	...	...	8	95	97	97	94	...	*75*
Saint Vincent and the Grenadines	...	...	...	...	8	100	100	100	100	...	*98*
Eastern Mediterranean											
Djibouti	...	60-79	79	100-249	11	51	69	69	68	65	*56*
Europe											
Bosnia and Herzegovina	...	...	...	...	...	20	58	65	52	...	...
Croatia	...	...	...	...	...	92	85	85	90	...	...
Monaco	...	...	...	...	...	100	98[f]	98	98	...	...
San Marino	...	...	...	...	5	...	100	100	100	...	...
Slovenia	...	...	...	<25	...	96	98	98	90	...	...
Tajikistan	...	...	...	100-249	...	69	82	74	97	...	...
The Former Yugoslav Republic of Macedonia	...	...	...	...	...	87	70	94	96	...	...
Turkmenistan	...	...	...	25-99	...	94	71	92	84	...	...
Yugoslavia	...	≥90	...	...	...	81	79	81	75	...	...
Western Pacific											
Cook Islands	...	...	...	...	...	94	100	100	100	80	*8*
Kiribati	...	...	...	...	7	87	86	100	89	78	*85*
Marshall Islands	...	...	...	...	...	88	56	52	36	9	...
Micronesia (Federated States of)	...	...	...	...	...	50	79	78	76	44	...
Nauru	...	...	...	...	...	93	74	74	...	...	...
Niue	...	...	...	...	...	100	100	100	100	...	...
Samoa	...	...	...	...	6	82	81	81	81	44	60
Tonga	...	...	...	...	3	96	100	100	87	68	40
Tuvalu	...	...	...	...	...	100	69	79	64	16	...
Vanuatu	...	...	...	...	7	84	77	77	66	47	66

[a] Figures in italics are the latest available and not for the year(s) specified.
[b] Figures refer to BCG, diphtheria-pertussis-tetanus (third dose), oral poliovirus (third dose), measles and tetanus toxoid.
[c] Figures refer to use of oral rehydration salts and/or recommended home fluid.
[d] In some countries measles immunization is given at, or later than, 12 months and up to 2 years.
[e] The three targets in WHO's strategy for health for all by the year 2000 relating to health status are: life expectancy at birth above 60 years; infant mortality rate below 50 per 1 000 live births; under-5 mortality rate below 70 per 1 000 live births.
[f] Diphtheria-tetanus only.
[g] Two doses only.
... Data not available or not applicable.

Table A3. Basic indicators

Estimates are obtained or derived from relevant WHO programmes or from responsible international agencies for the areas of their concern

| Member States | Annual number of reported cases for selected diseases | | | | | % of population with access to safe water 1988-91 | | % of population with access to adequate sanitation 1988-91 | |
	Tuberculosis 1993	Malaria 1992	Polio[a] 1993	Measles 1993	Neonatal tetanus 1993	Total	Rural	Total	Rural
WHO Member States meeting all three health-for-all targets[b]									
Africa									
Mauritius	...	...	0	88	0	96	92	94	96
Americas									
Argentina	14 041	643	0	1 555	5	65	17	69	35
Canada	...	...	0	187	0	...	...	...	...
Chile	...	...	0	1	1	86	...	83	20
Colombia	11 043	184 023	0	5 668	71	86	82	64	18
Costa Rica	...	6 951	0	579	0	93	86	97	94
Cuba	...	...	0	...	0	98	91	92	68
El Salvador	...	4 539	0	38	18	47	19	58	36
Jamaica	...	...	0	0	0	100	100	89	80
Mexico	...	16 170	0	169	97	76	68	50	17
Panama	...	727	0	90	2	83	66	84	68
Paraguay	...	1 289	0	2 066	29	35	24	62	67
Trinidad and Tobago	...	...	0	0	0	97	91	79	98
United States of America	25 313	1 087	0	281	0	...	...	...	...
Uruguay	689	...	0	16	0	75	5	61	65
Venezuela	...	21 416	0	20 244	15	89	89	92	70
Eastern Mediterranean									
Iran (Islamic Republic of)	22 470	76 971	107	4 616	12	89	75	71	35
Jordan	278	0	0	2 985	6	99	97	100	100
Kuwait	391	...	0	260	0	...	...	...	...
Lebanon	0	...	0	396	0	92	85	...	...
Oman	289	14 827	2	3 108	0	84	77	71	40
Saudi Arabia	2 386	19 623	2	3 182	35	95	74	86	30
Syrian Arab Republic	126	456	0	2 300	74	74	58	83	82
Tunisia	2 565	...	0	1 413	3	99	99	96	94
United Arab Emirates	327	3 605	0	745	0	95	...	77	22
Europe									
Albania	295	...	0	7	...	...	...	...	...
Austria	1 268	...	0	0	...	...	...	...	...
Belgium	1 503	...	0	...	...	...	...	...	...
Bulgaria	3 213	...	0	354	0	...	...	...	...
Denmark	419	...	0	115	0	...	...	...	...
Estonia	532	...	0	312	0	...	...	...	...
Finland	542	...	0	0	0	...	...	...	...
France	9 551	...	0	...	...	...	...	...	...
Germany	14 161	...	0	...	...	...	...	...	...
Greece	171	...	0	514	...	...	...	...	...
Hungary	4 209	...	0	39	0	...	...	...	...
Ireland	...	...	0	4 328	...	...	...	...	...
Israel	440	...	0	119	0	...	...	...	...
Italy	4 734	...	0	16 890	0	...	...	...	...
Latvia	1 646	...	0	54	...	...	...	...	...
Lithuania	1 895	...	0	249	0	...	...	...	...
Netherlands	1 579	...	7	468	0	...	...	...	...
Norway	...	...	0	7	0	...	...	...	...
Poland	16 828	...	0	1 410	0	...	...	...	...
Portugal	5 447	...	0	881	0	...	...	...	...
Romania	20 349	...	2	28 321	1	...	...	...	...
Spain	9 441	...	0	11 977	...	...	...	...	...
Sweden	672	...	0	25	0	...	...	...	...
Switzerland	...	...	0	...	0	...	...	...	...
United Kingdom	6 575	...	2	12 022	0	...	...	...	...

Member States	Annual number of reported cases for selected diseases					% of population with access to safe water 1988-91		% of population with access to adequate sanitation 1988-91	
	Tuberculosis 1993	Malaria 1992	Polio[a] 1993	Measles 1993	Neonatal tetanus 1993	Total	Rural	Total	Rural
South-East Asia									
Democratic People's Republic of Korea	...	...	...	...	...	...	...	...	...
Sri Lanka	6 573	399 349	5	242	5	60	55	50	45
Thailand	13 814	168 370	10	9 159	51	77	72	74	72
Western Pacific									
Australia	906	...	0	4 421	0	...	...	...	...
China	344 218	72 026	538	117 851	...	72	68	79	81
Japan	...	...	0	...	...	97	85	...	...
Malaysia	12 285	36 853	0	542	9	78	66	81	...
New Zealand	367	...	0	6	0	97	82	...	...
Philippines	178 134	110 457	15	...	343	82	79	69	62
Republic of Korea	...	...	0	...	...	97	96	100	100
Singapore	1 830	...	0	...	...	100	...	99	...
Viet Nam	52 994	212 000	452	12 015	333	24	21	17	13
WHO Member States not meeting all three health-for-all targets[b]									
Africa									
Angola	...	...	...	...	...	41	20	19	15
Benin	...	...	104	4 102	79	51	46	34	31
Burkina Faso	...	...	7	14 890	20	68	72	10	5
Burundi	4 677	...	5	23 869	13	57	54	49	47
Cameroon	2 404	...	30	14 171	345	48	27	74	64
Central African Republic	...	...	11	...	...	24	26	46	46
Chad	...	...	...	16 208	419	57	70	...	...
Congo	...	...	0	693	8	38	2	...	...
Côte d'Ivoire	...	...	...	...	...	76	81	60	62
Gabon	...	...	8	...	...	68	50	...	...
Ghana	...	...	19	31 220	8	52	35	42	32
Guinea	...	...	15	5 228	30	53	56	21	5
Guinea-Bissau	...	...	2	1 707	...	41	35	31	32
Kenya	20 451	...	...	...	...	49	43	43	35
Liberia	1 766	...	3	6 398	119	50	22	...	...
Madagascar	9 855	...	19	6 060	21	23	9	3	3
Malawi	17 105	...	0	3 614	16	56	50	84	81
Mali	...	...	26	10 595	40	41	38	24	10
Mauritania	...	...	16	5 754	3	66	65	...	...
Mozambique	...	...	1	5 506	37	22	17	20	11
Namibia	...	...	56	...	7	52	35	14	11
Niger	...	...	41	37 051	46	53	45	14	4
Nigeria	11 597	...	1 083	52 242	1 984	36	30	35	30
Rwanda	...	...	4	9 861	7	66	62	58	56
Senegal	...	...	2	14 693	63	48	26	55	36
Sierra Leone	2 691	...	5	2 288	99	37	37	58	49
Togo	...	...	3	2 966	25	60	53	23	10
Uganda	...	...	...	...	...	33	30	32	28
United Republic of Tanzania	31 827	...	2	16 592	53	49	45	64	62
Zaire	...	...	33	2 708	90	39	24	23	11
Zambia	...	...	8	8 256	26	53	28	37	12
Zimbabwe	...	...	0	5 902	1	84	80	40	22
Americas									
Haiti	...	13 457	0	...	...	39	33	24	16
Eastern Mediterranean									
Afghanistan	...	...	...	...	...	23	19	...	...
Pakistan	313	103 084	1 803	1 967	1 685	56	45	24	10
Somalia	...	...	...	...	...	37	29	18	5
Sudan	1 684	...	252	683	71	48	43	75	65
Yemen	...	29 320	58	601	8	36	30	65	60

Member States	Annual number of reported cases for selected diseases					% of population with access to safe water 1988-91		% of population with access to adequate sanitation 1988-91	
	Tuberculosis 1993	Malaria 1992	Polio[a] 1993	Measles 1993	Neonatal tetanus 1993	Total	Rural	Total	Rural
South-East Asia									
Bangladesh	54 001	115 660	233	5 443	720	84	81	31	26
Bhutan	100	28 900	0	495	0	34	30	13	7
Myanmar	12 019	125 710	44	2 288	107	32	...	36	35
Nepal	13 161	23 234	2	58	20	42	39	6	3
Western Pacific									
Cambodia	...	91 000	135	1 262	88	36	33	14	8
Lao People's Democratic Republic	826	41 787	7	1 083	11	36	33	21	8
Papua New Guinea	5 247	...	0	3 632	70	33	20	...	...
WHO Member States meeting at least one of the values above the health-for-all target[b]									
Africa									
Algeria	1 468	...	0	3 141	40	68	55	57	40
Botswana	...	...	0	4 608	0	90	88	88	85
Cape Verde	...	...	0	0	1	...	...	...	...
Lesotho	3 383	...	1	12	0	47	45	22	23
South Africa	88 319	...	0	12 808	16	...	...	...	...
Americas									
Bahamas	54	...	0	0	0	...	...	...	...
Barbados	2	...	0	0	0	...	...	...	...
Bolivia	...	24 486	0	2 702	21	52	27	26	13
Brazil	...	609 860	0	4 326	216	87	61	72	32
Dominican Republic	3 826	698	0	4 637	0	67	45	87	75
Ecuador	...	41 089	0	3 628	81	55	43	48	38
Guatemala	...	57 560	0	17	19	62	43	60	52
Guyana	80	39 702	0	0	0	...	...	...	...
Honduras	3 745	70 838	0	13	6	77	63	61	43
Nicaragua	2 798	26 866	0	339	7	54	21	...	...
Peru	...	54 922	0	1 730	120	56	10	57	20
Suriname	14	1 404	0	0	0	...	...	...	...
Eastern Mediterranean									
Bahrain	114	...	2	2	0	...	...	...	...
Cyprus	37	...	0	0	0	...	...	...	...
Egypt	3 416	...	150	2 874	1 277	90	86	50	26
Iraq	...	18 451	75	16 339	171	77	41	...	...
Libyan Arab Jamahiriya	735	...	0	733	0	97	80	98	85
Morocco	27 588	405	0	8 431	8	56	18	...	...
Qatar	200	...	0	27	0	...	...	...	...
Europe									
Armenia	...	...	0	206	...	...	...	...	...
Azerbaijan	2 954	...	70	584	...	...	...	...	...
Belarus	4 134	...	1	3 874	0	...	...	...	...
Czech Republic	1 864	...	0	13	0	...	...	...	...
Georgia	...	...	0	405	...	...	...	...	...
Iceland	...	...	...	39	...	...	...	...	...
Kazakhstan	9 992	...	1	3 297	0	...	...	...	...
Kyrgyzstan	...	...	0	3 825	...	...	...	...	...
Luxembourg	...	...	0	4	...	...	...	...	...
Malta	26	...	0	3	0	...	...	...	...
Republic of Moldova	1 938	...	1	863	0	...	...	...	...
Russian Federation	112 964	...	1	74 463	...	...	...	...	...
Slovakia	1 799	...	0	551	0	...	...	...	...
Turkey	...	18 676	18	34 285	46	78	63	...	...
Ukraine	19 964	...	5	23 452	0	...	...	...	...
Uzbekistan	7 227	...	68	3 353	0	...	...	...	...

Member States	Annual number of reported cases for selected diseases					% of population with access to safe water 1988-91		% of population with access to adequate sanitation 1988-91	
	Tuberculosis 1993	Malaria 1992	Polio[a] 1993	Measles 1993	Neonatal tetanus 1993	Total	Rural	Total	Rural
South-East Asia									
India	...	2 125 800	4 198	49 932	4 339	85	85	16	2
Indonesia	...	13 655[c]	26	58 238	566	51	43	44	36
Maldives	123	...	0	61	1	...	...	...	...
Mongolia	1 418	...	0	71	0	80	58	74	47
Western Pacific									
Brunei Darussalam	...	...	0	...		...	...	...	...
Fiji	183	...	0	143	0	...	...	...	...
Solomon Islands	...	153 359	0	...	...	...	...	...	...
WHO Member States for which insufficient data are available for life expectancy, infant mortality and under-5 mortality									
Africa									
Comoros	...	...	0	0	1	...	...	...	...
Equatorial Guinea	...	...	0	157	4	...	...	...	...
Eritrea	...	...	...	...	...	...	...	...	...
Ethiopia	...	...	...	...	...	...	...	...	...
Gambia	...	...	0	792	13	...	...	...	...
Sao Tome and Principe	...	...	0	88	5	...	...	...	...
Seychelles	...	...	0	0	0	...	...	...	...
Swaziland	...	...	0	6 942	2	...	...	...	...
Americas									
Antigua and Barbuda	...	...	0	0	0	...	...	...	...
Belize	34	5 341	0	0	0	...	...	...	...
Dominica	4	...	0	0	0	...	...	...	...
Grenada	...	...	0	0	0	...	...	...	...
Saint Kitts and Nevis	...	...	0	0	0	...	...	...	...
Saint Lucia	...	...	0	0	0	...	...	...	...
Saint Vincent and the Grenadines	...	...	0	0	0	...	...	...	...
Eastern Mediterranean									
Djibouti	...	...	0	37	0	...	...	...	...
Europe									
Bosnia and Herzegovina	...	...	0	70		...	...	...	...
Croatia	2 279	...	0	87	0	...	...	...	...
Monaco	...	...	0	...		...	...	...	...
San Marino	...	...	0	3	...	...	...	...	...
Slovenia	646	...	0	8	0	...	...	...	...
Tajikistan	652	...	14	5 045	...	...	...	...	...
The Former Yugoslav Republic of Macedonia	1 712	...	0	2 495	1	...	...	...	...
Turkmenistan	1 061	...	2	2 486	...	...	...	...	...
Yugoslavia		...	7	16 859	...	...	...	...	...
Western Pacific									
Cook Islands	7	...	0	3	0	...	...	...	...
Kiribati	122	...	0	116	2	...	...	...	...
Marshall Islands	61	...	0	...	...	...	...	...	...
Micronesia (Federated States of)	...	...	0	...	...	...	...	...	...
Nauru	...	...	0	...	...	...	...	...	...
Niue	1	...	0	0	0	...	...	...	...
Samoa	49	...	0	0	0	...	...	...	...
Tonga	32	...	0	...	...	...	...	...	...
Tuvalu	28	...	0	0	0	...	...	...	...
Vanuatu	...	13 330	0	...	...	...	...	...	...

[a] Cases were indigenous in all countries except for vaccine-associated (VA) and wild virus/imported (IM) cases in Albania (1 VA), Belarus (1 IM), Croatia (1 VA), Germany (1 VA), Italy (2 VA), Lithuania (2 VA), Poland (2 VA), Romania (8 VA), Russian Federation (2 VA), United Kingdom (1 IM), USA (2 VA, 1 IM) and Yugoslavia (3 VA).

[b] The three targets in WHO's strategy for health for all by the year 2000 relating to health status are: life expectancy at birth above 60 years; infant mortality rate below 50 per 1 000 live births; under-5 mortality rate below 70 per 1 000 live births.

[c] Java and Bali only; in the other islands 1.31 million clinical malaria cases were recorded in 1992.

... Data not available or not applicable.

Table B. Analytical tabulations

Indicator	Year	Unit	WHO Member States	Developed world			Developing world		
				Total	Developed market economies	Economies in transition	Total	Developing countries other than LDCSs	Least developed countries (LDCs)
1 Population	1993	millions	5 559	1 206	812	394	4 353	3 796	556
Growth rate per annum	1990-2015	%	1.5	0.5	0.5	0.5	1.7	1.6	2.6
2 Total fertility rate	1990-1995	per woman	3.3	1.9	1.8	2.2	3.8	3.4	6.0
3 Population under 15 years	1993	millions	1 783	255	157	98	1 529	1 283	246
Percentage of total population	1993	...	32.1	21.1	19.3	24.7	35.1	33.8	44.1
Growth rate per annum	1990-2015	%	0.8	0.1	0.1	0.2	0.9	0.6	2.2
4 Population aged 65 years and above	1993	millions	355	152	111	42	202	186	17
Percentage of total population	1993	...	6.4	12.6	13.7	10.6	4.6	4.9	3.0
Growth rate per annum	1990-2015	%	2.4	1.5	1.5	1.4	3.0	3.0	3.0
Elderly support ratio (65+/20-64)	1993	%	12.2	21.4	22.7	18.5	9.2	9.5	7.0
5 Median age of population	1993	years	24.6	33.9	35.0	31.7	22.1	22.7	17.7
6 Population in urban areas	1992	millions	2 391	884	624	260	1 507	1 394	113
Percentage of total population	1992	...	43.9	73.7	77.4	66.2	35.4	37.5	21.1
7 Population in agglomeration > 10 million	1990	millions	177	63	63	0	114	114	0
Percentage of urban population	1990	% urban population	7.7	7.2	7.2	...	8.1	8.1	...
Average annual growth rate	1990-2010	%	4.5	1.3	0.6	...	5.7	5.4	...
8 Gross domestic product (GDP)	1993	1988 US$ (billions)	20 863	16 920	15 419	1 501	3 943	...	...
Average annual growth rate	1983-1993	%	2.5	2.2	2.7	−2.3	4.0	...	...
Gross domestic product per capita	1993	1988 US$	3 793	14 030	18 989	3 810	918	...	...
External debt/GDP ratio	1990	%	...	...	...	...	31.4	...	62.8
9 Adult literacy rate, both sexes	1990	%	...	...	...	98	67	69	44
Literacy rate, females	1990	%	...	...	...	97	58	60	33
10 Gross primary enrolment ratio	1990	%	99.0	101.8	...	...	98.4	101.3	64.7
Percentage of drop-outs from primary education	1988	% new entrants	...	...	...	...	26.6	25.3	40.0
11 Higher enrolment/primary enrolment ratio	1990	%	10.5	31.5	...	...	5.7	6.0	2.4
12 Public education expenditure	1991	US$ (billions)	1 119	951	...	...	168	163	5
Percentage of gross national product	1991	...	5.1	5.3	...	...	4.1	4.1	3.3
13 Age and sex standardized death rate	1990-1995	per 100 000 population	930	569	493	743	1 036	933	1 706
14 Life expectancy at birth	1993	years	66	75	77	71	64	66	51
15 Crude death rate	1990-1995	per 100 000 population	930	970	939	1 035	919	821	1 588
16 Infant mortality rate	1993	per 1 000 live births	62	12	7	20	69	59	110
17 Under-5 mortality rate	1992	per 1 000 live births	96	10	9	21	104	87	179
18 0-4 death rate	1990	per 100 000 population	2 066	...	207	507	...	1 952	4 301
19 20-49 death rate, males	1990	per 100 000 population	343	...	201	414	...	321	753
20 20-49 death rate, females	1990	per 100 000 population	261	...	94	149	...	262	690
21 65-74 death rate	1990	per 100 000 population	3 599	...	2 529	3 577	...	3 985	5 444
22 75 years and above death rate	1990	per 100 000 population	10 849	...	9 220	10 987	...	11 999	14 137
23 Maternal mortality	1990	per 100 000 live births	370	26	11	42	420	349	735
24 Low birth weight	1990	% of live births	17	7	6	7	19	17	23
25 Prenatal care	1990	% of live births	64	98	96	100	59	63	45
26 Deliveries attended by trained personnel	1990	% of live births	60	99	99	98	55	61	30
27 ORS and/or RHF use rate[a]	1993	%	...	...	...	...	44	45	43
28 Access to safe water	1988-1991	%	...	...	...	...	70	73	49
29 Access to adequate sanitation	1988-1991	%	...	...	...	...	51	54	33
30 Health expenditure per capita	1990	US$	327	1 295	1 860	137	36	39	11
31 Public expenditure on defense per capita	1991	1987 US$	125	455	...	...	30	...	...

[a] Oral rehydration salts and/or recommended home fluid.
... Data not available or not applicable.

Index